Retina

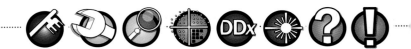

Rapid Diagnosis in Ophthalmology
Series Editors: Jay S. Duker MD, Marian S. Macsai MD
Associate Editor: Gary S. Schwartz MD

Anterior Segment
Bruno Machado Fontes, Marian S. Macsai
ISBN 978-0-323-04406-6

Lens and Glaucoma
Joel S. Schuman, Viki Christopoulos, Deepinder K. Dhaliwal,
Malik Y. Kahook, Robert J. Noecker
ISBN 978-0-323-04443-1

Neuro-ophthalmology
Jonathan D. Trobe
ISBN 978-0-323-04456-1

Oculoplastic and Reconstructive Surgery
Jeffrey A. Nerad, Keith D. Carter, Mark Alford
ISBN 978-0-323-05386-0

Pediatric Ophthalmology and Strabismus
Mitchell B. Strominger
ISBN 978-0-323-05168-2

Retina
Adam H. Rogers, Jay S. Duker
ISBN 978-0-323-04959-7

Commissioning Editor: Russell Gabbedy
Development Editor: Martin Mellor Publishing Services Ltd
Project Manager: Rory MacDonald
Design Manager: Stewart Larking
Illustration Manager: Merlyn Harvey
Illustrator: Jennifer Rose
Marketing Manager(s) (UK/USA): John Canelon/Lisa Damico

Series Editors: Jay S. **Duker** MD, Marian S. **Macsai** MD

Associate Editor: Gary S. **Schwartz** MD

Rapid Diagnosis in Ophthalmology
Retina

By
Adam H. Rogers MD

Assistant Professor of Ophthalmology, Tufts University School of Medicine,
Boston, MA, USA

Jay S. Duker MD

Director, New England Eye Center, Vitreoretinal Diseases and Surgery Service;
Professor and Chair of Ophthalmology, Tufts University School of Medicine,
Boston, MA, USA

Series Editors
Jay S. Duker MD

Director, New England Eye Center, Vitreoretinal Diseases and Surgery Service;
Professor and Chair of Ophthalmology, Tufts University School of Medicine,
Boston, MA, USA

Marian S. Macsai MD

Chief, Division of Ophthalmology, Evanston Northwestern Healthcare; Professor
and Vice-Chair, Department of Ophthalmology, Feinberg School of Medicine,
Northwestern University, Chicago, IL, USA

Associate Editor
Gary S. Schwartz MD

Adjunct Associate Professor, Department of Ophthalmology, University of
Minnesota, Minneapolis, MN, USA

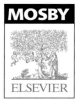

MOSBY

ELSEVIER

Mosby is an affiliate of Elsevier Inc.

First published 2008

ISBN 978-0-323-04959-7

British Library Cataloguing in Publication Data
A catalogue record for this book is available from the British Library

Library of Congress Cataloging in Publication Data
A catalog record for this book is available from the Library of Congress

Notice
Medical knowledge is constantly changing. Standard safety precautions must be followed, but as new research and clinical experience broaden our knowledge, changes in treatment and drug therapy may become necessary or appropriate. Readers are advised to check the most current product information provided by the manufacturer of each drug to be administered to verify the recommended dose, the method and duration of administration, and contraindications. It is the responsibility of the practitioner, relying on experience and knowledge of the patient, to determine dosages and the best treatment for each individual patient. Neither the Publisher nor the authors assume any liability for any injury and/or damage to persons or property arising from this publication.

The Publisher

Printed in China
Last digit is the print number: 9 8 7 6 5 4 3 2 1

Contents

Contents

12 Inflammatory Diseases

13 Infectious Diseases

Given the complexity and quantity of clinical knowledge required to correctly identify and treat ocular disease, a quick reference text with high quality color images represents an invaluable resource to the busy clinician. Despite the availability of extensive resources online to clinicians, accessing these resources can be time consuming and often requires filtering through unnecessary information. In the exam room, facing a patient with an unfamiliar presentation or complicated medical problem, this series will be an invaluable resource.

This handy pocket sized reference series puts the knowledge of world-renowned experts at your fingertips. The standardized format provides the key element of each disease entity as your first encounter. The additional information on the clinical presentation, ancillary testing, differential diagnosis and treatment, including the prognosis, allows the clinician to instantly diagnose and treat the most common diseases seen in a busy practice. Inclusion of classical clinical color photos provides additional assurance in securing an accurate diagnosis and initiating management.

Regardless of the area of the world in which the clinician practices, these handy references guides will provide the necessary resources to both diagnose and treat a wide variety of ophthalmic diseases in all ophthalmologic specialties. The clinician who does not have easy access to sub-specialists in Anterior Segment, Glaucoma, Pediatric Ophthalmology, Strabismus, Neuro-ophthalmology, Retina, Oculoplastic and Reconstructive Surgery, and Uveitis will find these texts provide an excellent substitute. World-wide recognized experts equip the clinician with the elements needed to accurately diagnose treat and manage these complicated diseases, with confidence aided by the excellent color photos and knowledge of the prognosis.

The field of knowledge continues to expand for both the clinician in training and in practice. As a result we find it a challenge to stay up to date in the diagnosis and management of every disease entity that we face in a busy clinical practice. This series is written by an international group of experts who provide a clear, structured format with excellent photos.

It is our hope that with the aid of these six volumes, the clinician will be better equipped to diagnose and treat the diseases that affect their patients, and improve their lives.

Marian S. Macsai and Jay S. Duker

The initial goal of this book was to create a concise, accessible manual with high quality photos of primarily common retinal diseases that a general ophthalmologist or retinal specialist encounter on a daily basis. The format was efficient and straightforward with a breakdown of diseases divided into key facts, clinical findings, ancillary testing, differential diagnosis, treatment and prognosis. Thus, the pertinent facts of a specific disease could be rapidly accessed without having to laboriously delve into a large textbook.

While I feel our primary goal has been achieved, the finished product exceeds the initial intent with the addition of more photographs and diseases covered. As I wrote the manuscript, I continued to add additional material that I felt was necessary to create a more complete book. Not only are basic retinal diseases now covered, but rare diseases that one may encounter potentially once in a five to ten year period are included.

By no means does this book encompass all diseases of the retina and choroid. That was never my intent. With the rapid pace at which new discoveries and advancements are made one must continue to remain up to date to fully ensure that their patients are receiving the most modern and efficacious treatment available. Nonetheless, this book will assist in the locating the diagnosis and rapidly familiarizing the physician with the disease at hand.

Adam H. Rogers

To Stephanie, Ben, Julia and David for their unwavering support during the writing of this book.

Adam H. Rogers

Dedication

Section 1

Diabetes

Non-proliferative Diabetic Retinopathy

Key Facts

- Diabetic retinopathy is the leading cause of legal blindness in persons aged 20–65 years in industrialized nations
- Occurs in both type 1 and type 2 diabetes
- Duration of disease and severity of hyperglycemia are greatest risk factors for developing retinopathy
- Hypertension, smoking, and hyperlipidemia are comorbid factors

Clinical Findings

- Microaneurysms and intraretinal hemorrhages
- Cotton wool spots
- Hard exudates
- Intraretinal microvascular abnormalities (IRMAs)
- Retinal capillary non-perfusion
- Macular edema
- Venous beading
- Stages
  - Minimal non-proliferative diabetic retinopathy (NPDR): rare microaneurysms • Mild to moderate NPDR: retinal microaneurysms and intraretinal hemorrhage with or without macular edema • Severe NPDR: over 20 intraretinal hemorrhages in all four quadrants of retina, venous beading in two or more quadrants, and IRMAs in one quadrant (4 : 2 : 1 rule)

Ancillary Testing

- Optical coherence tomography to evaluate for macular edema
- Fluorescein angiography identifies microaneurysms, areas of leakage to guide laser treatment and capillary non-perfusion

Differential Diagnosis

- Hypertensive retinopathy • Sickle cell retinopathy • Radiation retinopathy • Branch or central vein occlusion • Ocular ischemic syndrome • Idiopathic juxtafoveal telangiectasis • Arterial macroaneurysm • Anemia • Leukemia • Coats disease

Treatment

- Intensive blood glucose and blood pressure control, dietary modification and exercise under supervision of primary care physician

Prognosis

- 5–10% of all diabetic eyes will show progressive retinal disease each year
- 25% of those with type 1 diabetes will have diabetic retinopathy after 5 years of disease, 60% at 10 years, and 80% after 15 years
- In those with type 2 diabetes of duration <5 years, 40% taking insulin and 24% not on insulin will have retinopathy; this increases to 84% and 53%, respectively, at 19 years
- Eyes with severe NPDR have a 75% risk of developing proliferative diabetic retinopathy within 1 year
- Pregnancy and tighter blood glucose control may accelerate severity of diabetic retinopathy, necessitating a funduscopic examination every trimester

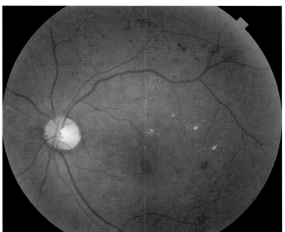

Fig. 1.1 Severe NPDR with dot and blot hemorrhages, microaneurysms, and mild hard exudate.

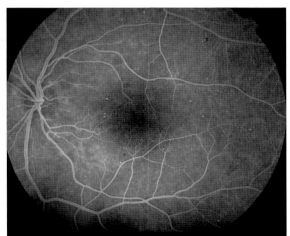

Fig. 1.2 Focal areas of hyperfluorescence from microaneurysms in an eye with mild NPDR.

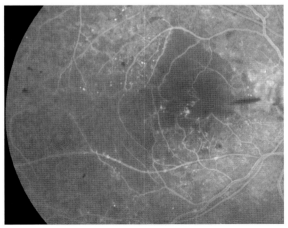

Fig. 1.3 Macular non-perfusion shown on fluorescein angiography in this eye with NPDR causing a decline in visual acuity to 20/80.

Clinically Significant Macular Edema

Key Facts

- Retinal thickening with or without hard exudate that involves or threatens the fovea
- Occurs from increasing permeability of retinal capillaries
- May cause vision loss in eyes with non-proliferative or proliferative diabetic retinopathy
- Risk of visual loss is greatest when fovea is involved or macular edema is diffuse
- Diagnosed by slit-lamp examination

Clinical Findings

- Retinal thickening at or within 500 μm of center of macula
- Hard exudates at or within 500 μm of center of macula with adjacent retinal thickening
- Retinal thickening measuring one disc area or more within one disc diameter of center of fovea

Ancillary Testing

- Optical coherence tomography measures macular edema and monitors response of retina to treatment
- Fluorescein angiography identifies microaneurysms and areas of leakage to guide laser treatment

Differential Diagnosis

- Hypertensive retinopathy
- Radiation retinopathy
- Branch or central retinal vein occlusion
- Idiopathic juxtafoveal telangiectasis
- Arterial macroaneurysm
- Diabetic retinopathy

Treatment

- Administered when clinically significant macular edema (CSME) present
- Focal laser photocoagulation applied as light small burns directly to leaking microaneurysms
- Grid laser photocoagulation is a grid-like pattern of light burns to a diffuse area of retinal edema
- Intravitreal triamcinolone acetonide 4 mg/0.1 mL administered when CSME unresponsive to laser
- Pars plana vitrectomy when taut posterior hyaloid or preretinal proliferation present

Prognosis

- Laser photocoagulation reduces risk of moderate visual loss by 50% compared with untreated eyes
- **Although a promising and effective treatment for CSME, intravitreal corticosteroids are limited by side effects:**
  - cataract formation • ocular hypertension • tachyphylaxis with repeated injections

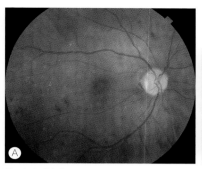

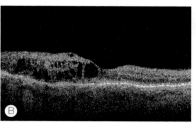

Fig. 1.4 (**A**) Foveal cysts are visible on close examination of the color image of this eye with CSME. (**B**) The intraretinal fluid is easily visible on optical coherence tomography.

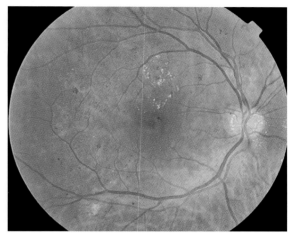

Fig. 1.5 CSME defined as hard exudate within 500 μm of the center of the fovea, with associated retinal thickening.

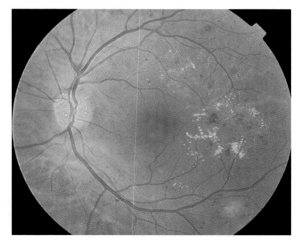

Fig. 1.6 CSME with retinal exudates, microaneurysms, and retinal fluid measuring one disc area or more within one disc diameter of the fovea.

Proliferative Diabetic Retinopathy

Key Facts

- More severe, advanced form of diabetic retinopathy
- Occurs when impaired retinal perfusion and ischemia induce retinal neovascularization on inner surface of retina and optic nerve
- The posterior vitreous hyaloid acts as a scaffold for new blood vessel growth
  - Vitreous hemorrhage occurs when neovascular fronds bleed, typically induced by hyaloid traction
  - Neovascular fronds eventually undergo fibrosis and traction, which may result in epiretinal membrane formation and retinal detachment

Clinical Findings

- Findings of non-proliferative diabetic retinopathy
- Neovascularization of the retina, optic nerve, and/or iris
- Preretinal fibrosis with or without retinal traction
- Neovascular glaucoma
- **High-risk characteristics present when:**
  - neovascularization occurs with vitreous hemorrhage
  - neovascularization at optic disc equals one-quarter to one-third of disc area even without vitreous hemorrhage

Ancillary Testing

- Ultrasound when vitreous hemorrhage prevents visualization of retina
- Fluorescein angiography to evaluate for areas of neovascularization or retinal capillary non-perfusion
- Optical coherence tomography to document epiretinal membrane or presence of clinically significant macular edema (CSME)
- Gonioscopy to identify neovascularization of iris and angle
- Applanation tonometry to measure for elevated IOP

Differential Diagnosis

- Sickle cell retinopathy
- Radiation retinopathy
- Ocular ischemic syndrome
- Familial exudative vitreoretinopathy
- Venous occlusive disease (branch and central retinal vein occlusion)
- Coats disease
- Eales disease

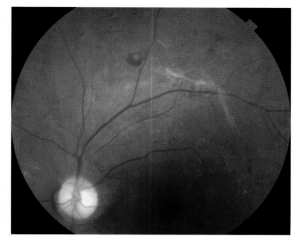

Fig. 1.7 A neovascular frond with early fibrosis is present along the superior temporal arcade.

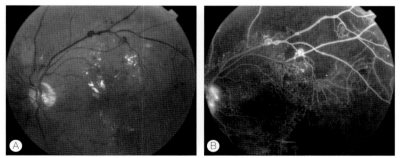

Fig. 1.8 Red-free photograph (**A**) and FA (**B**) of severe PDR with exudate, venous beading, intraretinal hemorrhage, neovascularization of the disc and extensive capillary nonperfusion.

Treatment

- Panretinal photocoagulation (PRP) when high-risk characteristics present
- Focal or grid laser should be performed if CSME present before PRP to minimize PRP-induced exacerbation of macular edema
- Pars plana vitrectomy with endolaser in non-clearing vitreous hemorrhage
- Anti–vascular endothelial growth factor injected into the vitreous 1 week before a planned procedure may be useful as adjunctive treatment to help clear vitreous hemorrhage before PRP or to induce regression of neovascularization before pars plana vitrectomy
  - Regression of neovascularization before surgery may limit intraoperative bleeding, making surgery technically less difficult
- Intensive blood glucose control under supervision of primary care physician

Prognosis

- Untreated proliferative diabetic retinopathy may lead to decreased vision from traction retinal detachment or progressive capillary non-perfusion
- PRP reduces risk of severe vision loss when high-risk characteristics present

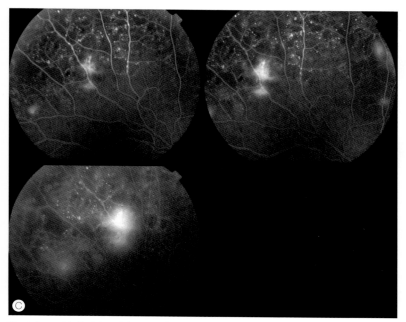

Fig. 1.8, cont'd Peripheral image of the FA (**C**) reveals leakage from neovascularization.

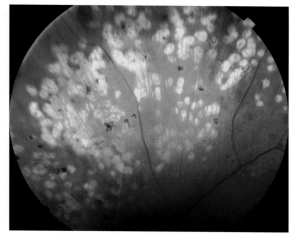

Fig. 1.9 Peripheral scars from pan retinal photocoagulation.

Diabetic Traction Retinal Detachment

Key Facts

- Advanced, severe form of proliferative diabetic retinopathy
- Regression of vascular component of neovascular frond with fibrotic proliferation
- Fibrosis and contraction of preretinal neovascular fronds induce retinal traction
- Formation of retinal breaks may occur from traction creating a rhegmatogenous detachment

Clinical Findings

- Preretinal fibrosis typically extending from optic nerve along vascular arcade
- Localized or total retinal detachment
- **Traction retinal detachments typically:**
  - taut • concave toward pupil • no evidence of shifting subretinal fluid
    - confined to the posterior pole
- Retinal breaks typically in posterior pole and difficult to visualize
- Capillary non-perfusion
- Neovascularization of iris and angle
- Neovascular glaucoma
- Preretinal or vitreous hemorrhage (may resolve by presentation)
- Hypotony from chronic retinal detachment
- All findings from non-proliferative and proliferative diabetic retinopathy may be present

Ancillary Testing

- Ultrasound when vitreous hemorrhage prevents visualization of retina
- Optical coherence tomography to determine if macula is detached
- Gonioscopy to evaluate for neovascularization of iris and angle
- Applanation tonometry to measure IOP

Differential Diagnosis

- Rhegmatogenous retinal detachment with proliferative vitreoretinopathy

Treatment

- Limited traction retinal detachments in peripheral retina that do not threaten macula should be observed
- Panretinal photocoagulation if previous laser has not been performed or is inadequate
- Pars plana vitrectomy with endolaser, membrane peel, and internal tamponade with gas or silicone oil when detachment threatens or involves fovea
- Intravitreal anti–vascular endothelial growth factor injected 1 week before vitrectomy surgery may make the surgery less complicated by inducing involution of any active neovascularization
- Control of blood glucose and blood pressure

Prognosis

- Vast majority of patients have a poor visual prognosis from the advanced stage of diabetic retinopathy, even if the traction detachment does not involve fovea
- Visual recovery after vitrectomy surgery is limited and depends on duration of macular detachment and severity of capillary non-perfusion

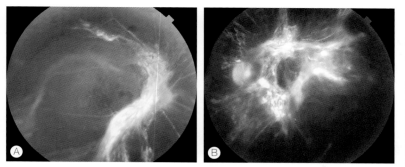

Fig. 1.10 (**A**) Right and (**B**) left eye of a female patient with advanced proliferative diabetic retinopathy and bilateral traction retinal detachments. Thick fibrosis is visible in the macula. A combined traction and rhegmatogenous retinal detachment is present in the right eye, with a retinal tear in the papillomacular bundle.

Section 2
Age-related Macular Degeneration

Non-exudative Age-related Macular Degeneration

Key Facts

- Leading cause of vision loss in people ≥65 years in developed countries
    - Non-exudative (dry) age-related macular degeneration (AMD) represents 80% of all cases of AMD • Causes nearly 20% of all vision loss in eyes with AMD • Vision decline occurs from photoreceptor dysfunction and loss primarily from geographic atrophy • Prevalence of dry AMD 13–20% in persons >40 years (depending on epidemiologic study), with increasing incidence associated with advanced age • Progressive • Bilateral • Unknown etiology • Age, family history, smoking, light-colored irides are greatest risk factors

Clinical Findings

- Drusen
- Pigment clumping
- Focal atrophy of retinal pigment epithelium (RPE)
- Geographic atrophy

Ancillary Testing

- Fluorescein angiography to evaluate choroidal neovascularization (CNV)
    - Drusen stain with mild, early fluorescence that fades in later frames • Window defect in areas of RPE atrophy
- **Optical coherence tomography:**
    - undulation of RPE layer represents drusen • thinning of retina in areas of atrophy

Differential Diagnosis

- Neovascular AMD • Myopic degeneration • Pattern dystrophy • Angioid streaks • Stargardt disease • Best's disease • Acute multifocal posterior placoid epitheliopathy • Central serous retinopathy (chronic and inactive) • Plaquenil toxicity

Treatment

- **For patients with intermediate or advanced dry AMD, daily vitamin supplements including:**
    - vitamin C 500 mg • vitamin E 400 IU • beta-carotene 15 mg • zinc 80 mg • copper 2 mg (validated based on the findings of the Age-related Macular Degeneration Eye Disease Study, AREDS)
- Observation with dilated funduscopic examination should be performed every 6 months (sooner if patients complain of metamorphopsia or decreasing visual acuity)

Prognosis

- Natural history of disease in patients >65 years with mild dry AMD observed over 3 years showed a new non-exudative or exudative lesion in 9% at 1 year, 16% at 2 years, and 24% at 3 years
- If neovascular AMD in one eye, risk of developing CNV in fellow eye is 7–10% per year
- Antioxidants plus zinc decrease risk of progression to advanced AMD by 25% (based on AREDS results)

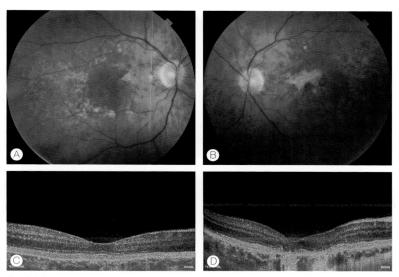

Fig. 2.1 Drusen temporally and geographic atrophy centered in the macula are visible in the (**A**) right and (**B**) left eye of this female patient with dry AMD. Disruption of the photoreceptor layer is present in both eyes (**C,D**) but more severe in the left eye (**D**) as imaged on ultra high-resolution optical coherence tomography. In (**D**), there is almost complete loss of the photoreceptor layer, with increased reflectivity into the choroid layer. Visual acuity measures 20/30 in the right and 20/80 in the left eye due to the geographic atrophy.

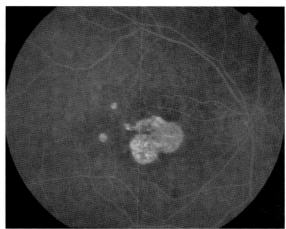

Fig. 2.2 Window defect on fluorescein angiography in an eye with advanced dry AMD and geographic atrophy.

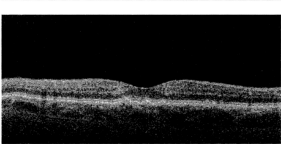

Fig. 2.3 Drusen imaged on Stratus optical coherence tomography appear as mild undulations of the RPE.

Neovascular Age-related Macular Degeneration

Key Facts

- 20% of all cases of age-related macular degeneration (AMD)
- Causes 80% of vision loss in all eyes with AMD
- Often associated with abrupt decline in visual acuity
- Vascular endothelial growth factor (VEGF), along with other factors, stimulates growth of choroidal neovascularization (CNV)
- Cascade of events initiating VEGF release is unknown
- May be unilateral, with a tendency toward bilaterality

Clinical Findings

- Subretinal fluid
- Intraretinal fluid
- Sub–retinal pigment epithelium (RPE) fluid
- Subretinal hemorrhage
- Drusen
- Exudate
- Fibrosis
- Disciform scar
- Breakthrough vitreous hemorrhage

Ancillary Testing

- Fluorescein angiography (FA) is the gold standard for evaluating and classifying CNV
  - Classic lesions have early, well-defined hyperfluorescence with late leakage
    - Occult membranes show speckled hyperfluorescence that may be well defined or have vague borders • Serous pigment epithelial detachments show pooling of fluorescein in sub-RPE space with an adjacent occult CNV
    - Lesions can be classified as subfoveal (under the geometric center of the foveal avascular zone, FAZ), juxtafoveal (1–199 μm from FAZ center), or extrafoveal (≥200 μm from FAZ center) • The Treatment of AMD with Photodynamic Therapy study group defined CNV as predominately classic (≥50% of lesion is classic), minimally classic (<50% of lesion is classic with the remainder occult), and occult without classic lesions (pure occult lesion without a classic component)
- Indocyanine green (ICG) angiography tends to stain CNV as a plaque in occult and classic CNV
  - ICG most useful when identifying either a focal area of leakage (hot spot) or CNV adjacent to serous pigment epithelial detachment in occult CNV, otherwise FA more beneficial
- Optical coherence tomography (OCT) images the CNV as a hyper-reflective yellow-red extension of the RPE extending into the retina
  - Intraretinal and subretinal fluid present in active disease • OCT useful when evaluating response of retina to treatment • Retinal fluid collections absent in well-treated CNV but return when CNV reactivated
- Ultrasound when vitreous hemorrhage present to evaluate for retinal detachment

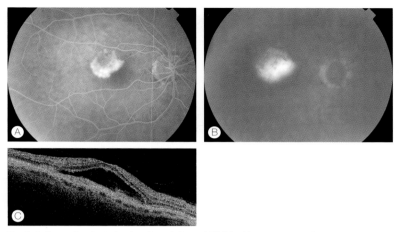

Fig. 2.4 A predominately classic subfoveal CNV without an occult component is evident with (**A**) early, well-defined hyperfluorescence and (**B**) late leakage. (**C**) A neurosensory detachment is present on OCT.

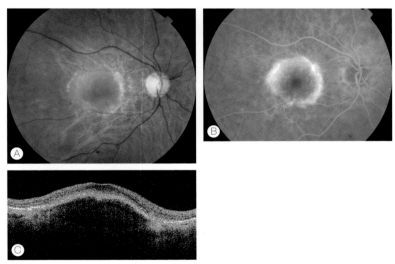

Fig. 2.5 A fibrovascular pigment epithelial detachment (occult CNV) viewed as (**A**) a color image and (**B**) with speckled hyperfluorescence on FA. (**C**) On OCT, there is elevation of the RPE layer with a normal foveal contour.

Differential Diagnosis

- Central serous retinopathy • Myopic degeneration • Idiopathic juxtafoveal telangiectasia • Ocular histoplasmosis syndrome • Diabetic retinopathy • Idiopathic polypoidal choroidal vasculopathy

Treatment

- Ranibizumab (Lucentis) for both classic and occult CNV
- Bevacizumab (Avastin) as an off-label treatment
- Photodynamic therapy (PDT) with verteporfin (Visudyne) for predominately classic subfoveal CNV, with or without intravitreal corticosteroids
- Laser photocoagulation to well-defined juxtafoveal and extrafoveal CNV
- Observation for disciform scars
- Pars plana vitrectomy for non-clearing breakthrough vitreous hemorrhage

Prognosis

- Untreated CNV disease leads to disciform scar and 20/200 or worse visual acuity in nearly all cases
- Minimally classic and occult without classic lesions treated with ranibizumab injected into the vitreous cavity every 4 weeks for 24 months showed an overall average improvement in vision of 7.2 letters on an Early Treatment Diabetic Retinopathy Study (ETDRS) chart compared with a 10.4 letter loss in untreated eyes at 2 years compared with control eyes
- In a trial comparing ranibizumab versus PDT with verteporfin, ranibizumab proved clinically efficacious in eyes with predominately classic, subfoveal CNV
  - At 12 months, ranibizumab-treated eyes gained on average 8.5 (0.3-mg dose) and 11 (0.5-mg dose) letters on an ETDRS chart compared with an average loss of 9.5 letters in the PDT treatment group
- PDT was the first laser to treat subfoveal CNV without significant retinal damage
  - It is effective against predominately classic CNV • In eyes with predominately classic subfoveal CNV treated with PDT, 67% lost <15 letters compared with 39% in eyes assigned to placebo; no statistically significant differences in visual acuity were noted in minimally classic and occult lesions
- The Submacular Surgery Trials showed no benefit of surgical removal of subfoveal CNV compared with observation
- In juxtafoveal CNV treated with thermal laser photocoagulation at 5 years, 48% of treated eyes compared with 62% of untreated eyes lost six or more lines; recurrent lesions occurred in 54% of treated eyes
- In extrafoveal CNV treated with thermal laser photocoagulation, 52% of treated eyes compared with 61% of untreated eyes lost six or more lines at 5 years, with a 47% recurrent rate of CNV

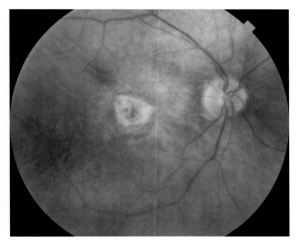

Fig. 2.6 Disciform scar formation in an eye with end stage neovascular AMD.

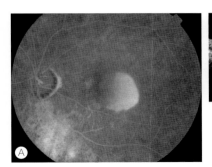
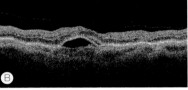

Fig. 2.7 Pooling of fluorescein dye into the sub-RPE space in a serous pigment epithelial detachment imaged on (**A**) FA and (**B**) OCT.

Idiopathic Choroidal Neovascularization

Key Facts

- Abnormal proliferation of blood vessels that originate in the choroid, break through Bruch's membrane, and remain under or extend through the retinal pigment epithelium (RPE) layer
- No clinical evidence of other etiologies of choroidal neovascularization (CNV)
- Women affected more than men
- Usually unilateral
- Occurs in third to fifth decades
- Presents with decreased visual acuity and metamorphopsia

Clinical Findings

- Decreased visual acuity (and metamorphopsia)
- Subretinal or intraretinal hemorrhage
- Intraretinal and subretinal fluid
- Lipid exudation
- Hyperplasia of RPE cells
- Fibrous scar tissue

Ancillary Testing

- Fluorescein angiography delineates the CNV with early hyperfluorescence and late leakage
  - Idiopathic CNV is usually a well-defined classic lesion without an occult component
- Optical coherence tomography images both intraretinal and subretinal fluid collections
  - The CNV is imaged as a hyper-reflective extension of the RPE layer extending underneath the retina
- Indocyanine green (ICG) will define the CNV but is useful only if hemorrhage is blocking the lesion, otherwise ICG is of minimal value in diagnosis and treatment

Differential Diagnosis

- Age-related macular degeneration (AMD)
- Myopic degeneration
- Ocular histoplasmosis syndrome
- Punctate inner choroidopathy
- Angioid streaks

Treatment

- Intravitreal anti–vascular endothelial growth factor (VEGF)
- Photodynamic therapy
- Oral prednisone
- Submacular surgery

Prognosis

- Natural history of untreated, subfoveal idiopathic CNV disease is variable, with vision tending to decrease
- Photodynamic therapy has shown some success in treating subfoveal CNV in limited uncontrolled case series
- Intravitreal anti-VEGF injections are gaining in popularity and may be the most effective form of treatment
- Submacular surgery results from multiple case reports show high recurrence rates
- Oral prednisone may be of limited value when used as monotherapy
- Overall, visual outcome better in eyes with idiopathic CNV compared to eyes with AMD

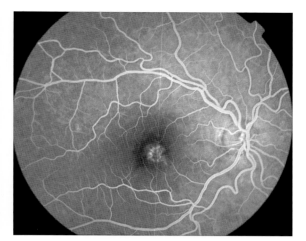

Fig. 2.8 A 54-year-old woman presented with 20/200 vision from a subfoveal, classic CNV on fluorescein angiography in 2003. She was treated with photodynamic therapy twice, with a final visual acuity of 20/80. Note that there are no drusen, RPE changes, or atrophy that would be found in AMD.

Myopic Degeneration

Key Facts

- Progressive degeneration of retina from a pathologic increase in axial length
- May lead to legal blindness
- Usually occurs in eyes with >6 D of myopia
- Highest prevalence in Asian people
- Women are affected twice as often as men
- Prevalence is about 2.1% in the USA
- Inherited as autosomal dominant or recessive trait or may occur sporadically
- May be associated with Ehlers–Danlos, Stickler, and Marfan syndromes

Clinical Findings

- Lattice degeneration
- Posterior staphyloma (ectasia of scleral wall)
- Tilted disc
- Temporal crescent or halo of atrophy surrounding optic disc
- Atrophy of retinal pigment epithelium (RPE) in macula
- Prominent choroidal vessels
- Choroidal neovascularization (CNV)
- Lacquer cracks
- Förster–Fuchs spot (hyperpigmented scar from regressed CNV)
- Vitreous syneresis
- Vitreous detachment

Ancillary Testing

- Fluorescein angiography to evaluate for CNV
- Window defect present in areas of RPE atrophy and lacquer cracks
- Optical coherence tomography can follow intraretinal or subretinal fluid collections from CNV; this information may be used to evaluate success of CNV treatment
- Ultrasound to confirm presence of posterior staphyloma

Differential Diagnosis

- Age-related macular degeneration
- Angioid streaks
- Ocular histoplasmosis syndrome

Treatment

- Intravitreal anti–vascular endothelial growth factor for subretinal CNV
- Photodynamic therapy for eyes with subfoveal CNV
- Argon laser photocoagulation for juxtafoveal and extrafoveal CNV

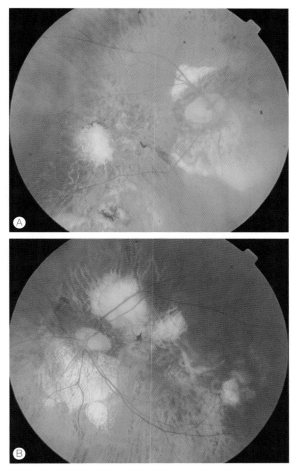

Fig. 2.9 The (**A**) right and (**B**) left eye of a patient with myopic degeneration. Both photographs show tilting of the optic nerve head, scattered macular and peripapillary atrophy, attenuation of the retinal arterioles, and RPE hyperplasia. The retina outside of the macula in the right eye (A) is slightly out of focus from the presence of a posterior staphyloma.

Myopic Degeneration (Continued)

Prognosis

- Pathologic myopia is a leading cause of blindness, with vision loss occurring from progressive atrophy or CNV formation
- Limited case series report that intravitreal bevacizumab (Avastin) may be effective in maintaining or improving visual acuity
- Verteporfin (Visudyne) for myopic CNV is effective at 1 year, with 72% of treated eyes compared with 44% of placebo-treated eyes losing fewer than eight letters at 12 months
  - At 2 years, the statistically significant benefit was no longer present—36% of verteporfin-treated eyes and 51% of placebo-treated eyes lost fewer than eight letters
- Laser photocoagulation effective at eliminating juxtafoveal or extrafoveal CNV but leads to eventual atrophy that may spread into the fovea over time, leading to diminished visual acuity
- Myopic eyes at greater risk for retinal detachment

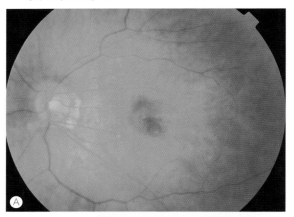

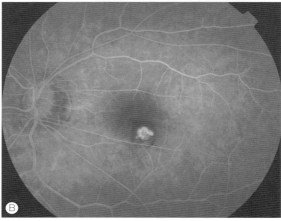

Fig. 2.10 (**A**) Color photograph and (**B**) accompanying fluorescein angiogram of a female patient with CNV from myopic degeneration. Note the pigmented spot at the fovea, with surrounding subretinal hemorrhage.

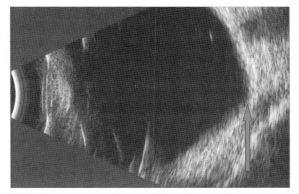

Fig. 2.11 An ultrasound of a patient with myopia, showing a posterior staphyloma.

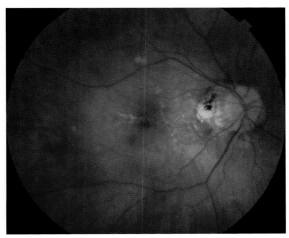

Fig. 2.12 Lacquer cracks course through the fovea of an eye with myopic degeneration. The four blurred specks in the vitreous are from asteroid hyalosis.

Angioid Streaks

Key Facts

- Unknown etiology
- Occurs from breaks in a calcified Bruch's membrane
- No sex or race predilection
- Bilateral
- Pseudoxanthoma elasticum the most common cause (50% of cases), followed by Ehlers–Danlos syndrome, Paget disease, and sickle cell hemoglobinopathies
- Vision loss occurs from formation of choroidal neovascularization (CNV) secondary to abnormal vessels growing through the breaks in Bruch's membrane
- Minor trauma can induce retinal hemorrhage

Clinical Findings

- Jagged, vessel-like reddish brown streaks deep to the retina that radiate from the optic disc in both eyes
- Peripapillary atrophy
- CNV
- Subretinal hemorrhage from CNV or minor blunt ocular trauma
- Optic nerve drusen
- Peau d'orange (mottling pigmentation of macula) in pseudoxanthoma elasticum
- Punched-out peripheral chorioretinal atrophy in pseudoxanthoma elasticum
- Plucked chicken appearance on skin of antecubital, neck, periumbilical, and inguinal regions in pseudoxanthoma elasticum

Ancillary Testing

- Fluorescein angiography (FA) to delineate angioid streaks when clinical signs are subtle
  - Hyperfluorescence of streaks varies based on amount of surrounding atrophy of retinal pigment epithelium
  - FA also identifies CNV when present; the CNV may be classic or occult
- Streaks on indocyanine green angiography are hyperfluorescent and more numerous and prominent than those imaged with FA
- Optical coherence tomography to evaluate intraretinal and subretinal fluid collections in active CNV
- Skin biopsy (pseudoxanthoma elasticum)
- Hemoglobin electrophoresis (sickle cell disease)
- Elevated serum alkaline phosphatase levels, bone x-ray, or bone scan (Paget disease)

Differential Diagnosis

- Age-related macular degeneration
- Pathologic myopia
- Choroidal rupture from trauma
- Ocular histoplasmosis syndrome

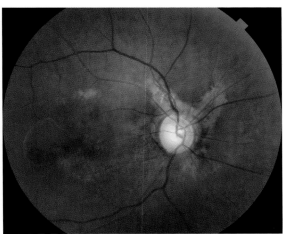

Fig. 2.13 Angioid streaks radiating from the disc in this eye show atrophy with hemorrhage present in the macula from a CNV.

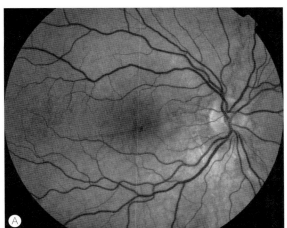

Fig. 2.14 (**A**) Angioid streaks are well delineated on red-free imaging and appear as vessels at the level of the choroid radiating out from the optic disc. (**B**) The angioid streaks stain with fluorescein.

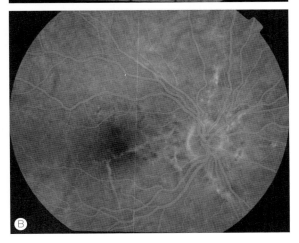

Treatment

- Angioid streaks without CNV require observation
- No effective treatment exists for subfoveal CNV
- Laser photocoagulation can be considered for juxtafoveal and extrafoveal CNV
- Photodynamic therapy with verteporfin (Visudyne) is ineffective
- Anti–vascular endothelial growth factor injected into vitreous cavity may be effective in maintaining visual acuity

Prognosis

- Angioid streaks without CNV are asymptomatic
- Poor visual prognosis for eyes with subfoveal CNV—no effective treatment exists

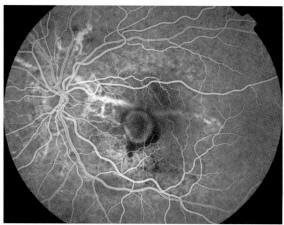

Fig. 2.15 A hyperfluorescent, ring-shaped choroidal neovascular membrane with surrounding blockage from hemorrhage is present, causing decline in visual acuity to 20/200 in this eye with angioid streaks.

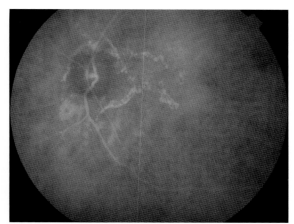

Fig. 2.16 Angioid streaks delineated in an eye after indocyanine green administration.

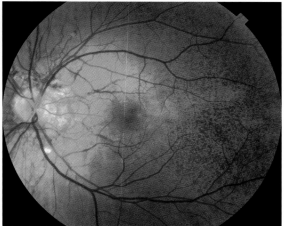

Fig. 2.17 Peau d'orange appearance is visible in the temporal aspect of the macula in this patient with angioid streaks and pseudoxanthoma elasticum.

Section 3

Vascular Obstructions

Branch Retinal Vein Occlusion

Key Facts
- Common cause of acute visual loss or visual field deficit
- Typically unilateral but may be bilateral in 5–10% of patients
- Men and women equally affected
- Most often occurs in elderly persons
- More common than central retinal vein occlusion
- Hypertension and arteriosclerosis are the major associations

Clinical Findings
- Decreased visual acuity
- Visual field defect corresponding to area of venous occlusion
- Intraretinal hemorrhage in the distribution along the obstructed retinal vein, with the apex of the hemorrhage at an arteriovenous crossing
- Macular edema
- Capillary non-perfusion and macular ischemia
- Retinal neovascularization
- Vitreous hemorrhage
- Collateral vessel formation in chronic disease

Ancillary Testing
- Fluorescein angiography (FA) to evaluate capillary non-perfusion and areas of retinal ischemia
- Optical coherence tomography to evaluate and monitor macular edema

Differential Diagnosis
- Diabetic retinopathy
- Hypertensive retinopathy
- Idiopathic juxtafoveal telangiectasia
- Radiation retinopathy
- Ocular ischemic syndrome

Treatment
- Laser treatment is guided by the Branch Retinal Vein Occlusion Study Group
- **Grid laser for macular edema:**
  - apply to eyes with 20/40 or worse vision for ≥3 months with intact foveal circulation
  - delay treatment if the macular hemorrhage is too dense to enable photocoagulation or evaluate retinal circulation on FA
  - withhold if decreased vision is due to capillary non-perfusion
- Panretinal photocoagulation to the peripheral non-perfused retina as visualized on FA when retinal neovascularization is present
- Intravitreal corticosteroids in eyes with macular edema, either as a primary treatment or in eyes refractory to grid laser photocoagulation
- Intravitreal anti–vascular endothelial growth factor (VEGF) therapy for macular edema, either as a primary treatment or in eyes refractory to grid laser photocoagulation
- Sheathotomy during pars plana vitrectomy to sever the common sheath shared by the arteriole and vein at the level of the obstruction to free the artery from compressing the vein

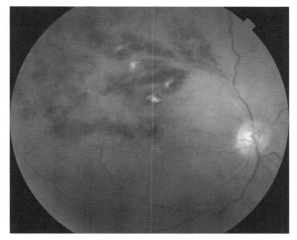

Fig. 3.1 Thick intraretinal hemorrhage along the superior temporal arcade extending into the fovea, with occasional cotton wool spots, in this color photograph of a BRVO.

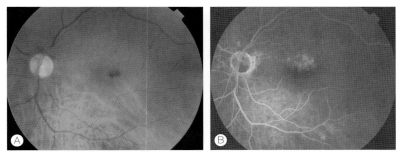

Fig. 3.2 A limited BRVO involving the fovea, with (**A**) intraretinal hemorrhage and (**B**) late leakage on FA.

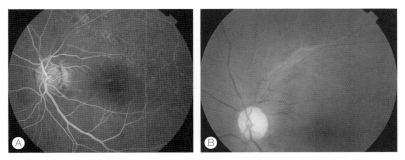

Fig. 3.3 Chronic BRVO with extensive vascular remodeling and shunt vessels along the superior temporal arcade. (**A**) The vascular changes do not involve the fovea on FA. (**B**) The occluded vein is sclerotic.

Branch Retinal Vein Occlusion (Continued)

Prognosis

- If the branch retinal vein occlusion (BRVO) occurs outside the macula, visual acuity is not affected
- **In eyes in which the macular circulation is affected by the BRVO:**
  - one-third will spontaneously improve to 20/40 or better
  - two-thirds will have decreased vision from macular edema, macular ischemia, thick macular hemorrhage, or vitreous hemorrhage
- Grid laser for macular edema increases visual improvement by two Snellen lines in 65% of treated eyes versus 37% of untreated eyes
- Panretinal photocoagulation in eyes with neovascularization reduces the risk of vitreous hemorrhage (29% in treated versus 61% in untreated eyes)
- Intravitreal corticosteroids, intravitreal anti-VEGF, and sheathotomy are all based on individual case reports—they have not been tested in randomized clinical trials to date

SECTION 3 • Vascular Obstructions

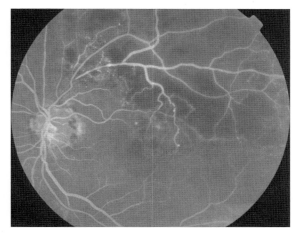

Fig. 3.4 Prominent capillary non-perfusion in the superior temporal quadrant that extends to the superior edge of the fovea in a BRVO that is more chronic in nature. The intraretinal hemorrhage has cleared, and capillary shunt vessels are present in the macula crossing the median raphe.

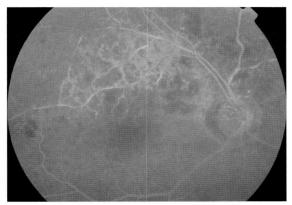

Fig. 3.5 Enlargement of the foveal avascular zone, causing decreased vision to 20/100. Note that there is no leakage in the macula as seen in Fig. 3.2. Grid laser was not performed.

Central Retinal Vein Occlusion

Key Facts

- Common retinal vascular disorder
- Occurs more often in persons over age 50
- Thrombosis of the central retinal vein at the level of the lamina cribrosa causes the central retinal vein occlusion (CRVO)
- Venous occlusion elevates venous pressure, resulting in stagnation of arterial blood flow and ultimate retinal hypoxia damaging the retina
- Associated with hypertension and diabetes
- Glaucoma is a common associated ocular disease
- May be categorized as either ischemic or non-ischemic
- Non-ischemic CRVO is more common, occurring in 75% of all cases
- Bilateral in 10% of patients

Clinical Findings

- Intraretinal hemorrhage with dilated and tortuous retinal veins in all four quadrants • Cotton wool spots • Optic disc swelling • Macular edema • Capillary non-perfusion • Neovascularization of retina or iris • Neovascular glaucoma • Vitreous hemorrhage • Relative afferent pupillary defect (RAPD) in ischemic CRVO • Venous collateral vessels at optic nerve (late finding)

Ancillary Testing

- Pupillary examination to evaluate for RAPD • Gonioscopy for evaluating the iris and angle for neovascularization • Fluorescein angiography is limited in early CRVO from blockage from retinal hemorrhage but can evaluate retinal circulation, non-perfusion, and retinal neovascularization • Electroretinogram may show a decreased b : a ratio

Differential Diagnosis

- Ocular ischemic syndrome • Diabetic retinopathy • Hypertensive retinopathy • Radiation retinopathy • Carotid cavernous or dural sinus fistula

Treatment

- Medically treat any underlying diabetes and hypertension
- Treat any underlying glaucoma
- Panretinal photocoagulation (PRP) of the peripheral retina when neovascularization of the iris, angle, or retina is present
  - PRP before formation of neovascularization is not beneficial and is advised only if there is considerable ischemia and close follow-up is not possible
- Focal laser photocoagulation is beneficial in reducing macular edema but has not been proven beneficial in improving visual acuity
- Intravitreal corticosteroids and intravitreal anti-VEGF injections have shown benefit in limited case reports

Prognosis

- About 34% of all eyes with perfused CRVO convert to non-perfused within 3 years
- Iris or angle neovascularization is found in about 16% of eyes
  - Increasing retinal vascular non-perfusion and decreasing visual acuity are the strongest predictors
- A natural history study published by the Central Vein Occlusion Study Group reported that initial visual acuity is the main predictor of final visual outcome

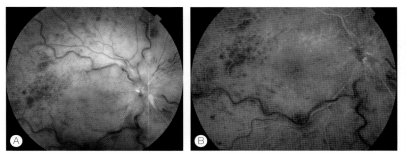

Fig. 3.6 (**A**) Color photograph and (**B**) FA of a central vein occlusion with disc swelling, dilated and tortuous veins, intraretinal hemorrhage in four quadrants, and macular edema. The arterioles are of normal caliber and unaffected.

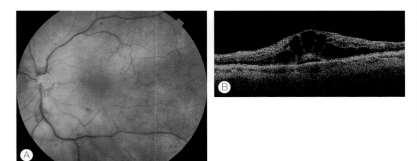

Fig. 3.7 (**A**) Non-ischemic CRVO with minimal intraretinal hemorrhage and dilated but not tortuous retinal veins. (**B**) Cystoid macular edema is present on the optical coherence tomography as black, hyporeflective intraretinal spaces.

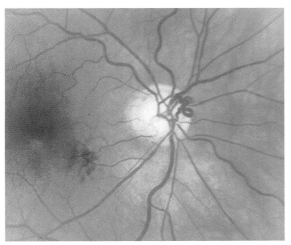

Fig. 3.8 Shunt vessel on the optic nerve in an eye with a resolved central vein occlusion.

Branch Retinal Artery Occlusion

Key Facts

- Rare event occurring less frequently than central retinal artery occlusion
- Men affected more commonly than women
- Most commonly occurs in sixth and seventh decades
- Right eye affected more commonly than the left eye
- Temporal retina more commonly affected than nasal retina
- Embolus is the most common cause
- **Risk factors include:**
  - diabetes • hypertension • hyperlipidemia • cardiac valvular disease • carotid artery disease • smoking
- Giant cell arteritis may be the etiology in 1–2% of cases

Clinical Findings

- Central visual acuity may be diminished or normal
- Visual field loss occurs in the area corresponding to the retinal ischemia
- Pupils may be normal or show a relative afferent defect
- **Acute clinical findings:**
  - retinal whitening and edema in area of ischemia • embolus
- **Chronic clinical findings:**
  - retinal whitening will resolve even if recanalization of the obstructed artery does not occur • loss of nerve fiber layer in area of ischemia, which may not be evident on physical examination • sheathing of the arteriole in the area of previous obstruction • arteriolar collaterals

Ancillary Testing

- Visual field test
- Fluorescein angiography shows diminished flow in the area of the obstructed arteriole, with delayed filling in the adjacent veins supplied
  - Late frames in the angiogram may show staining of the arteriole at the point of obstruction
- Carotid ultrasound to evaluate for carotid stenosis
- Cardiac echography to evaluate for cardiac and aortic source of emboli
- **Systemic medical evaluation of other etiologies should be considered in younger patients and includes:**
  - giant cell arteritis • pancreatitis • sickle cell disease • amniotic fluid embolus • systemic clotting disorders • homocystinuria • Kawasaki disease

Differential Diagnosis

- Central retinal artery occlusion • Cotton wool spot • Inflammatory or infectious chorioretinitis

Treatment

- No proven ocular therapy exists • Digital massage and anterior paracentesis may dislodge the embolus to a more distal arteriole, but each maneuver is rarely performed given the low success rate • Stroke work-up by the neurology service and prophylaxis with systemic anticoagulation should be instituted immediately, especially in elderly patients • Discontinue smoking and oral contraceptives • Intravenous or oral corticosteroids should be started if giant cell arteritis is suspected

Prognosis

- Visual field defects are permanent • Most patients retain 20/40 or better visual acuity unless the fovea is affected • Neovascularization uncommon

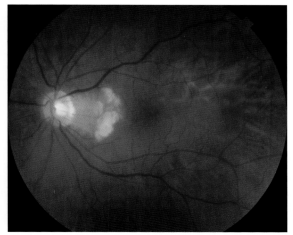

Fig. 3.9 Retinal whitening from retinal ischemia due to an embolus lodged at the bifurcation of the central retinal artery at the optic disc.

Cilioretinal Artery Occlusion

Key Facts

- A cilioretinal artery is present in 15–30% of the population
- Accounts for ≤5% of all arterial obstructions
- **Three variants are identified:**
  - isolated cilioretinal artery obstruction (40–45% of cases)
  - cilioretinal artery and central retinal vein occlusion (CRVO) (40%)
  - cilioretinal artery obstruction with anterior ischemic optic neuropathy (AION) (15%)

Clinical Findings

- **Isolated cilioretinal artery occlusion:**
  - decreased visual acuity • retinal whitening along the pathway of the artery
- **Combined cilioretinal artery and CRVO:**
  - decreased visual acuity • retinal whitening along the pathway of the artery
  - optic disc swelling • diffuse intraretinal hemorrhage
- **Combined cilioretinal artery and AION:**
  - swelling with hyperemia or pallor of optic disc • decreased visual acuity

Ancillary Testing

- Embolic work-up (rare with venous occlusion) including carotid and cardiac ultrasound
- Erythrocyte sedimentation rate for giant cell arteritis
- C-reactive protein for giant cell arteritis
- History and physical examination to evaluate for headaches, joint pain, scalp tenderness, scalp nodules, diminished or absent temporal artery pulse, and weight loss, which would indicate giant cell arteritis as the etiology
- Temporal artery biopsy

Differential Diagnosis

- CRVO
- Central retinal artery occlusion
- Branch retinal artery occlusion
- AION
- Hypertensive retinopathy
- Diabetic retinopathy
- Ocular ischemic syndrome

Treatment

- Systemic steroids when giant cell arteritis suspected or confirmed

Prognosis

- **Isolated cilioretinal artery occlusion:**
  - good visual prognosis • 90% of eyes improve to 20/40 or better vision
- **Combined cilioretinal artery and CRVO:**
  - good visual prognosis • acts similar to a non-ischemic CRVO • 70% or more achieve 20/40 or better • neovascularization rare
- **Combined cilioretinal artery and AION:**
  - poor visual outcome • visual acuity 20/400 to light perception

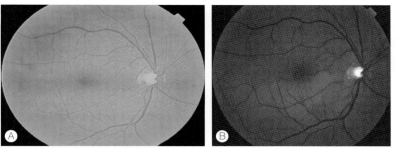

Fig. 3.10 (**A**) Color and (**B**) red-free photograph of a cilioretinal artery occlusion. Retinal whitening is present and more prominent in the red-free photograph. An embolus is visible in the cilioretinal artery, where it emerges from the optic nerve head on red-free imaging.

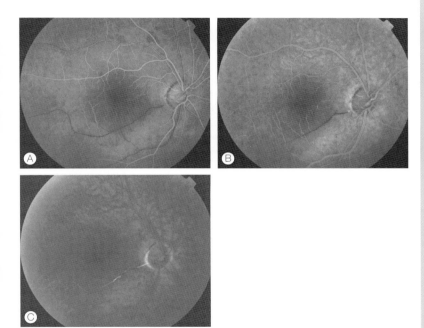

Fig. 3.11 (**A**) Early, (**B**) middle, and (**C**) late phase fluorescein angiogram of the same eye in Fig. 3.10, showing delayed perfusion through the cilioretinal artery. There is poor perfusion in the retina supplied by this vessel. Retrograde perfusion of the artery is present in the late frame of the angiogram.

Central Retinal Artery Obstruction

Key Facts

- Abrupt, painless loss of vision from diminished flow through the central retinal artery
- Occur at the central retinal artery or the ophthalmic artery
- Most common in elderly adults in the seventh decade
- Occurs in 1 in 10 000
- Men affected more than women
- Bilateral in 1–2% of cases
- Thrombus at the level of the lamina cribrosa is the most common cause
- Embolus seen in about 20% of eyes
- Giant cell arteritis occurs in 1–2% of cases
- Dissecting aneurysm is a rare cause
- In younger adults, central retinal artery obstruction may occur from migraine, coagulation disorders, hemoglobinopathies, or optic disc drusen

Clinical Findings

- Decreased visual acuity
- Relative afferent pupillary defect
- **Acute clinical findings:**
  - retinal whitening focused in the macula • cherry red spot at the fovea • narrow retinal arteries • visible red blood cell columns in the arteries (boxcarring) • patent cilioretinal artery (25% of eyes) • neovascularization of the iris (20%)
- **Chronic clinical findings:**
  - re-establishment of arterial circulation • loss of retinal whitening • narrowing of retinal arterioles • absence of visible nerve fiber layer • optic nerve pallor • optic disc collaterals • neovascular glaucoma • neovascularization of optic disc (2% of eyes)

Ancillary Testing

- Fluorescein angiography shows delay in retinal arteriolar filling in the acute setting
  - Delayed choroidal filling implies ophthalmic artery obstruction or carotid artery stenosis • The angiogram will revert to normal with re-establishment of arteriolar circulation
- Electroretinogram (ERG) with decreased b wave and normal a wave
  - With improved retinal blood flow, the ERG may normalize
- Visual fields may show a residual temporal island
  - In the presence of a patent cilioretinal artery, a small central island may remain
- Carotid ultrasound to evaluate for carotid artery disease
- Transthoracic or transesophageal cardiac ultrasound to evaluate for valvular disease or embolic source, especially in patients younger than 50
- Erythrocyte sedimentation rate for giant cell arteritis

Differential Diagnosis

- Commotio retina
- Multiple branch retinal artery obstructions
- Viral retinitis
- Cilioretinal artery obstruction

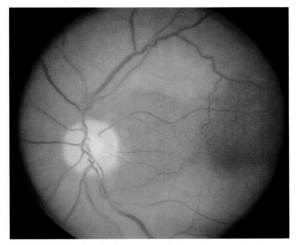

Fig. 3.12 Central retinal artery occlusion with a patent cilioretinal artery. The patient has a small central island with 20/40 vision, because the ischemia has spared the fovea.

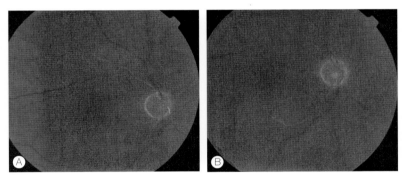

Fig. 3.13 (**A**) Middle and (**B**) late phase angiograms of a patient with a central retinal artery occlusion. Severe delay in arteriolar filling is present, with the leading edge of dye visible only to the level of the fovea at 5 min.

Treatment

- If performed, treatment must be instituted immediately; however, it is of uncertain efficacy
- Systemic corticosteroid treatment should be initiated immediately if giant cell arteritis is suspected or confirmed, to protect against vision loss in the second eye
- Digital massage for 10–15 s to increase the IOP, followed by release in an attempt to dislodge the embolus
- Carbogen administration (95% oxygen, 5% carbon dioxide) or rebreathing into a paper bag
- Anterior chamber paracentesis to abruptly lower IOP to advance the embolus
- Intravenous acetazolamide to lower IOP
- Panretinal photocoagulation with or without intravantreal anti–vascular endothelial growth factor when neovascularization is present
- Intraarterial or intravenous systemic clot dissolving medications in select, acute cases

Prognosis

- Visual acuity typically ranges from counting fingers to light perception
- Light perception visual acuity may be associated with an ophthalmic artery obstruction or giant cell arteritis
- Neovascularization of the iris occurs in 18% of eyes on average 4–5 weeks after obstruction
- A small central island with preserved visual acuity to the 20/20 level may be seen with perfusion of fovea in eyes with a patent cilioretinal artery

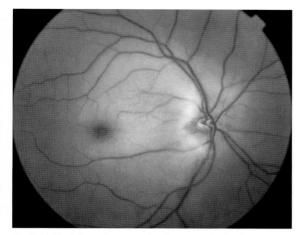

Fig. 3.14 Red-free photograph of a central retinal artery occlusion with diffuse retinal edema and ischemia present as retinal whitening.

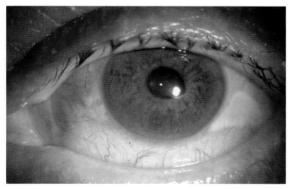

Fig. 3.15 Neovascularization of the iris with associated neovascular glaucoma is present in an eye with a central retinal artery occlusion. Intravitreal anti–vascular endothelial growth factor successfully induced regression of the abnormal iris vessels; however, the angle remained closed, with persistent elevated IOP.

Coats Disease

Key Facts

- Idiopathic
- Congenital
- Occurs in early childhood
- Males affected in 80% of cases
- Monocular in 80% of cases
- No inheritance pattern

Clinical Findings

- Severe visual loss
- Leukocoria
- Dilated capillaries
- Grape-like clusters of microaneurysms
- Sheathing of vessels
- Fusiform dilation of retinal blood vessels, resembling light bulbs
- Venous beading
- Capillary dropout and non-perfusion
- Lipid exudation that gravitates toward the macula
- Vitreous cells
- Strabismus
- **Chronic findings include:**
  - exudation
  - non-rhegmatogenous retinal detachment
  - macular fibrosis
  - iris neovascularization
  - cataract
  - neovascular glaucoma

Ancillary Testing

- Fluorescein angiography to delineate areas of leakage for treatment and to evaluate capillary non-perfusion
- Ultrasonography to evaluate for absence of calcification to rule out retinoblastoma
- CT with and without contrast to evaluate for absence of calcification to rule out retinoblastoma

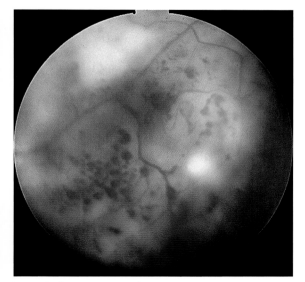

Fig. 3.16 Capillary non-perfusion with subretinal exudate and bulb-like fusiform dilatation of the retinal arterioles and mild venous dilation in Coats disease.

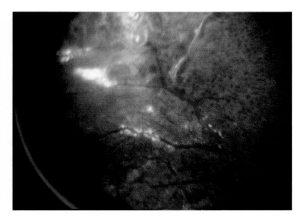

Fig. 3.17 Coats disease similar to figure 3.16, but with less retinal exudate.

Differential Diagnosis

- Branch retinal vein occlusion
- Diabetic retinopathy
- Idiopathic juxtafoveal telangiectasia
- von Hippel disease
- Rhegmatogenous retinal detachment
- Eales disease
- Vasculitis
- Collagen vascular disorders
- Radiation retinopathy
- Capillary hemangioma
- Pars planitis
- **Leukocoria:**
  - retinoblastoma
  - toxocariasis
  - retinopathy of prematurity
  - familial exudative vitreoretinopathy
  - persistent fetal vasculature
  - congenital cataract
  - incontinentia pigmenti
  - Norrie disease

Treatment

- Aggressive treatment with laser photocoagulation and/or cryotherapy to areas of leaking microaneurysms directly or in a scattered pattern
- Multiple treatments often needed
- Pars plana vitrectomy and scleral buckle may be considered for exudative detachments

Prognosis

- Lipid deposition in the fovea is irreversible and correlates with poor visual outcome
- The greater the area of vascular involvement, the more guarded the prognosis
- Late recurrences can occur, so patients require long-term follow-up

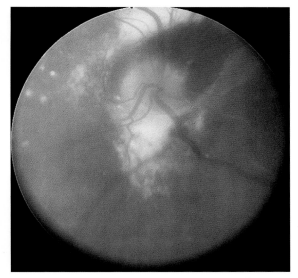

Fig. 3.18 Exudative retinal detachment in chronic Coats disease.

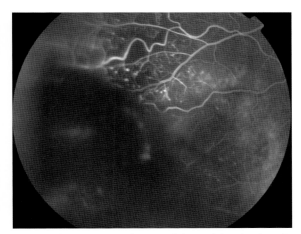

Fig. 3.19 Fluorescein angiogram of the peripheral retina of a teenaged girl with a history of exudative retinal detachment from Coats disease repaired with a scleral buckle. Note the microaneurysms and capillary non-perfusion.

Idiopathic Juxtafoveal Telangiectasia

Key Facts
- Idiopathic • Onset in fifth or sixth decade • Unilateral or bilateral
- Clinically divided into three subgroups
  - Unilateral cases have a male sex predilection similar to that seen in Coats disease (group 1) • Bilateral cases have no sex predilection (groups 2 and 3)
    - Group 3 is an occlusive form of the disease with some patients showing an inherited component

Clinical Findings
- **Group 1:**
  - Unilateral telangiectatic blood vessels temporal to the fovea • Exudate may be minimal or prominent with a circinate pattern • Cystoid macular edema (CME)
- Group 2
  - Bilateral and symmetric • Telangiectatic vessels are temporal to the fovea
    - Dilated retinal venules at right angles drain the telangiectatic capillaries
    - Minimal or absent CME • Absence of lipid exudate • Focal atrophy
    - Retinal pigment epithelial hyperplasia forms along venules • Crystalline deposits • Choroidal neovascularization (CNV)
- Group 3
  - Bilateral • Central nervous system vasculopathy

Ancillary Testing
- **Fluorescein angiography (FA):**
  - group 1 shows the telangiectatic vessels in the early frames with late parafoveal leakage; no capillary occlusion is present • group 2 eyes show the telangiectatic vessels more prominently on FA than on clinical examination, with late staining • group 3 eyes show bilateral occlusive disease on FA, with enlargement of the foveal avascular zone and mild late leakage
- Neuroimaging (CT, MRI) in group 3 patients may show cerebral infracts

Differential Diagnosis
- Diabetes • Branch retinal vein occlusion • Radiation retinopathy • Pars planitis • Tapetoretinal dystrophy • Retinal arterial macroaneurysm • Sickle cell retinopathy

Treatment
- Laser photocoagulation to the telangiectatic vessels in group 1 cases may stabilize or improve vision • Laser photocoagulation is of limited value in group 2, because there is usually no CME or exudate • Photodynamic therapy in eyes with subfoveal CNV • Intravitreal corticosteroids or anti–vascular endothelial growth factor injections may be considered but may be of limited value

Prognosis
- **Group 1:**
  - variable clinical course • patients may remain asymptomatic for many years
    - vision may fluctuate from 20/25 to 20/40 • severe visual loss may occur with extensive exudation
- **Group 2:**
  - variable visual acuity depends on presence of atrophy and CNV • reading vision in one eye may persist for years
- **Group 3:**
  - variable visual acuity based on extent of parafoveal occlusive disease

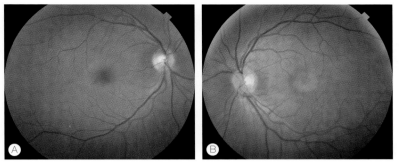

Fig. 3.20 The (**A**) right and (**B**) left macula of a woman with idiopathic juxtafoveal telangiectasia. Note the fine telangiectatic changes at the temporal edge of the fovea in both eyes.

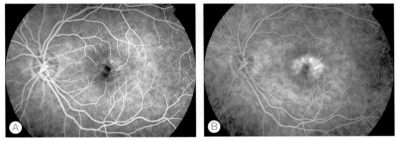

Fig. 3.21 Active leakage in the (**A**) arteriovenous and (**B**) late frames of the fluorescein angiogram from the left eye in Fig. 3.20B.

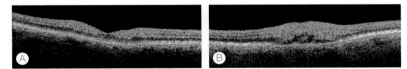

Fig. 3.22 A normal foveal contour in the right eye (**A**) with mild macular thickening from subretinal fluid in the left eye (**B**) in the optical coherence tomography images from the eyes in Fig. 3.20.

Radiation Retinopathy

Key Facts

- Changes in retina vasculature and optic nerve induced by radiation exposure
  - Risk of retinopathy increases with doses >3400 rad and fractional doses >200 rad • Comorbid factors include diabetes and hypertension • Typically a latent period of at least 6 months between radiation exposure and development of ocular disease exists • Disease may be categorized as similar to diabetes with non-proliferative and proliferative phases

Clinical Findings

- Microaneurysms • Retinal vascular telangiectasia • Exudates • Perivascular sheathing • Intraretinal hemorrhages • Cotton wool spots • Macular edema • Retinal arteriole occlusion • Intraretinal microvascular abnormalities • Venous beading • Neovascularization of retina, disc, and iris • Vitreous hemorrhage • Traction retinal detachment • Choroidal neovascularization • Optic nerve atrophy • Optic nerve edema (papillopathy) • Neovascular glaucoma

Ancillary Testing

- Fluorescein angiography to evaluate for capillary non-perfusion, leakage from microaneurysms, and neovascularization • Optical coherence tomography to identify macular edema • Visual field to document visual field loss from optic nerve injury

Differential Diagnosis

- Diabetic retinopathy • Branch retinal vein occlusion • Central retinal vein occlusion • Hypertensive retinopathy • Coats disease • Idiopathic juxtafoveal telangiectasia • Anterior ischemic optic neuropathy • Papilledema • Optic neuritis

Treatment

- Focal and/or grid laser photocoagulation for macular edema • Panretinal photocoagulation for proliferative disease with neovascularization of retina, optic disc, or iris • Intravitreal corticosteroids for macular edema not responsive to focal laser • Pars plana vitrectomy for non-clearing vitreous hemorrhage or traction retinal detachment • No proven treatment for radiation papillopathy

Prognosis

- Depends on extent of radiation damage to retina and optic nerve as well as extent of capillary occlusion

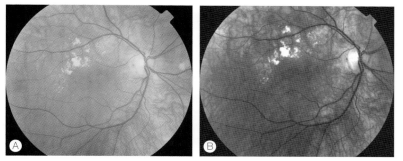

Fig. 3.23 (**A**) Color and (**B**) red-free photographs of microaneurysms and exudate of a patient with radiation retinopathy.

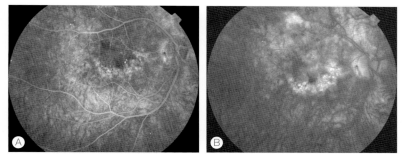

Fig. 3.24 Fluorescein angiogram of the same patient in Fig. 3.23, showing hyperfluorescence from (**A**) microaneurysms and (**B**) late cystoid macular edema.

Sickle Cell Retinopathy

Key Facts

- Chronic retinal vascular changes induced by genetic abnormalities in hemoglobin production
- Intravascular sickling, thrombosis, hemolysis, and hemostasis occur from altered red blood cells leading to the ocular changes
- Proliferative sickle cell retinopathy occurs most often in Hb SC disease followed by Sickle cell thalassemmia (SThal) and Sickle cell disease (HbSS)
- Visual deficits occur secondary to macular ischemia
- Severity of systemic illness does not directly correlate with ocular manifestations
- Bilateral

Clinical Findings

- Arteriolar occlusion
- Salmon patch hemorrhage (intraretinal hemorrhage after peripheral retinal arterial occlusion)
- Refractile deposits (hemosiderin left from reabsorbed hemorrhage)
- Black sunburst lesions (retinal pigment epithelium hyperplasia)
- Small red spots on optic disc
- Angioid streaks (6% of AS and SS disease)
- Peripheral retinal neovascularization (sea fan)
- Vitreous hemorrhage
- Traction and rhegmatogenous retinal detachment

Ancillary Testing

- Sickle cell solubility test (sickle cell preparation) is a screening tool to identify the presence of hemoglobin S; however, it does not differentiate between the heterozygote (Hb AS) and homozygote (Hb SS) states
- Hemoglobin electrophoresis is a definitive test done after a positive sickle cell solubility test
- Fluorescein angiography to evaluate macular circulation and peripheral retinal neovascularization
- Ultrasound when vitreous hemorrhage prevents visualization of retina

Differential Diagnosis

- Diabetic retinopathy
- Retinopathy of prematurity
- Familial exudative vitreoretinopathy
- Central retinal vein occlusion
- Branch retinal vein occlusion
- Ocular ischemic syndrome
- Branch retinal artery occlusion
- Hyperviscosity syndromes
- Carotid cavernous fistula
- Posterior uveitis
- Pars planitis
- Rhegmatogenous retinal detachment

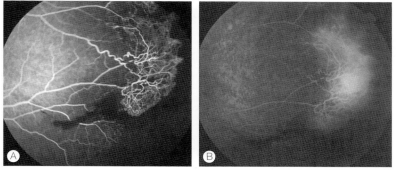

Fig. 3.25 Fluorescein angiogram sequence of the (**A**) middle and (**B**) late frames of peripheral retinal neovascularization (sea fan). There is blockage of fluorescence from the preretinal hemorrhage that is more visible in (A).

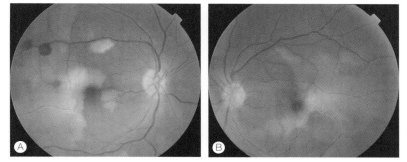

Fig. 3.26 A patient in a sickle cell crisis, with an acute, bilateral arteriolar occlusion. The ischemic retina is white.

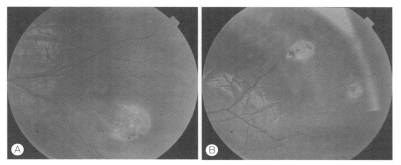

Fig. 3.27 Peripheral retinal pigment epithelial changes in an eye with sickle cell retinopathy.

Treatment

- Peripheral scatter laser photocoagulation to avascular peripheral retina when active neovascularization is present
  - Laser photocoagulation to close feeder vessels of neovascular fronds is not performed, because it may lead to hemorrhage and retinal breaks
- Areas of peripheral neovascularization that have autoinfarcted do not require peripheral scatter laser photocoagulation
- Pars plana vitrectomy for non-clearing vitreous hemorrhage and for retinal detachment
  - Encircling scleral buckles have been reported to cause anterior segment ischemia and should be used with caution

Prognosis

- Visual outcome variable and depends primarily on extent of macular ischemia
- Most patients maintain good visual acuity

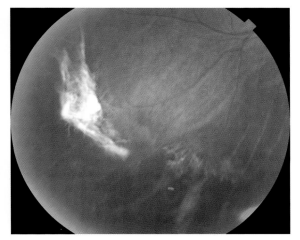

Fig. 3.28 An involuted peripheral sea fan visible as a white area of preretinal fibrosis occurring from autoinfarction.

Hypertensive Retinopathy

Key Facts

- Changes in retina, choroid, and optic nerve occurring with elevation of systemic arterial hypertension
- Most cases are chronic with changes in the retinal vasculature
- Occurs in about 15% of patients with hypertension
- Bilateral
- Men and women equally affected
- No racial predilection

Clinical Findings

- Arteriovenous nicking at crossing of retinal arteriole and vein
- Retinal arteriolar narrowing (most common finding)
- Cotton wool spots
- Nerve fiber layer hemorrhage
- Microaneurysms
- Macular edema
- Exudation
- Elschnig spots
- Neurosensory detachment
- Disc edema

Ancillary Testing

- Measurement of blood pressure

Differential Diagnosis

- Diabetic retinopathy
- Radiation retinopathy
- Vogt–Koyanagi–Harada disease
- Venous occlusive disease
- Ocular ischemic syndrome
- Hyperviscosity syndromes

Treatment

- Refer to primary care physician for treatment of chronic systemic arterial hypertension
- Immediate referral to emergency department for cases of acute systemic arterial hypertension

Prognosis

- Correction of blood pressure will lead to the resolution of acute clinical findings (disc edema, macular edema, and neurosensory detachment) within 2 weeks
  - More chronic findings of arteriolar narrowing and arteriovenous nicking rarely resolve
- Vision loss is rare unless chronic ischemia to the macula persists

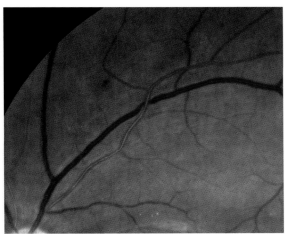

Fig. 3.29 Indentation of the vein at an arteriovenous crossing site (arteriovenous nicking) is present in an eye with mild hypertensive retinopathy. Note the mild venous dilation and narrowing of the arterioles.

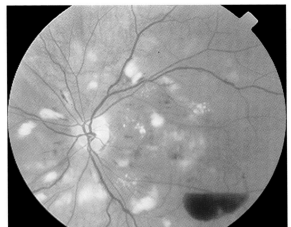

Fig. 3.30 Severe hypertensive retinopathy in a woman with advanced renal failure.

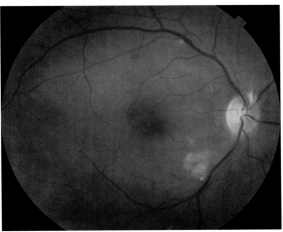

Fig. 3.31 Multiple cotton wool spots and narrowing of arterioles in an eye with hypertensive retinopathy.

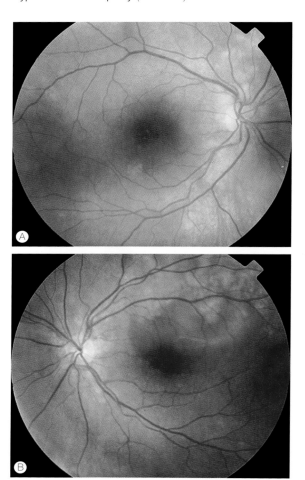

Fig. 3.32 (**A**) Right and (**B**) left eye of a woman with pregnancy-induced hypertension from pre-eclampsia. Focal yellow choroidal lesions are visible superior to the optic nerve in the right and along the superior temporal arcade in the left eye. In the left eye, subretinal fluid is visible. The fluid and yellow spots resolved with delivery.

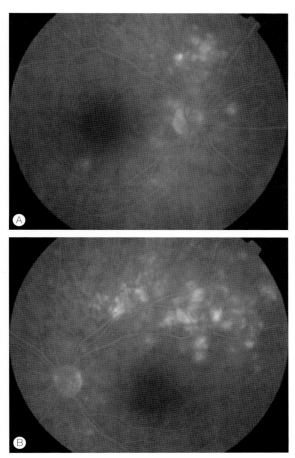

Fig. 3.33 Fluorescein angiography of the eyes from Figure 3.32 shows active leakage from the choroidal lesions of the (**A**) right and (**B**) left eye, as well as leakage from the disc.

Ocular Ischemic Syndrome

Key Facts

- Diminished ocular blood flow from severe carotid or ophthalmic artery stenosis
  - 90% stenosis of the vascular supply is required • Typically monocular
  - Occurring in men ≥65 years • Affected patients tend to have severe concomitant cardiovascular disease

Clinical Findings

- Slow visual loss occurring over weeks to months • Orbital ache • Prolonged visual recovery following exposure to bright light • Conjunctival injection • Corneal edema • Anterior chamber cellular response and flare • Iris neovascularization • Spontaneous arterial pulsations • Narrowing of retinal arterioles • Dilated veins, typically without tortuosity • Cherry red spot • Cotton wool spots • Midperipheral dot and blot hemorrhages • Neovascularization of the optic disc, retina, or iris • Low or normal IOP from ciliary body hypoperfusion • Neovascular glaucoma

Ancillary Testing

- **Signs of ocular ischemic syndrome in fluorescein angiography:**
  - choroidal filling that is delayed and patchy, lasting >5 s • a visible leading edge of dye in retinal arterioles • arteriovenous transit times >10 s
  - Arteriolar staining may be present
- Diminished a and b waves on electroretinogram
- Gonioscopy to identify neovascularization of the angle
- Carotid ultrasound to evaluate for significant carotid artery stenosis
- Color Doppler imaging to evaluate ocular blood flow and to assess reversal of blood flow in advanced cases

Differential Diagnosis

- Diabetic retinopathy • Central retinal vein occlusion • Giant cell arteritis • Hypertensive retinopathy • Takayasu arteritis • Blood dyscrasia • Arteriovenous malformation • Cavernous sinus or dural sinus fistula

Treatment

- Panretinal photocoagulation (PRP) when retinal or iris neovascularization is present • Carotid endarterectomy for 70–99% carotid artery stenosis decreased the rate of stroke in symptomatic patients—26% in medically treated patients compared with 9% in patients treated with endarterectomy (the North American Symptomatic Carotid Endarterectomy Trial) • Intravitreal anti-VEGF may be beneficial as adjunct treatment to PRP when iris neovascularization is present

Prognosis

- Visual prognosis better in milder cases, but there is a poor prognosis with more advanced stages of ocular ischemic syndrome • Elevated IOP may occur after carotid endarterectomy with improved ciliary body perfusion and increased aqueous production • PRP is successful in eradicating iris neovascularization in about one-third of all eyes • Affected patients have higher risk of cardiovascular events • 5-year mortality is around 40%

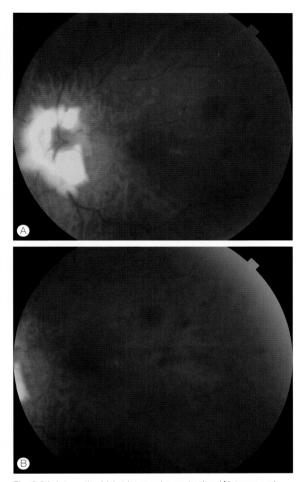

Fig. 3.34 Intraretinal blot hemorrhage in the (**A**) temporal macula and (**B**) midperipheral retina in an eye with ocular ischemic syndrome. Visual acuity measures 20/80. Carotid ultrasound measured a 90% stenosis, and the patient underwent carotid endarterectomy without change in clinical examination or visual acuity. A myelinated nerve fiber layer is present around the optic disc.

Retinal Arterial Macroaneurysm

Key Facts
- Occurs more frequently in women than men • Usually occurs in sixth and seventh decades • Hypertension is a major risk factor • Most common presentation is vision loss

Clinical Findings
- Focal, saccular dilatation of a retinal arteriole occurring within the first three orders of bifurcation • Intraretinal, subretinal, subhyaloid, and/or vitreous hemorrhage • Macular edema • Lipid exudation, often in a circinate pattern

Ancillary Testing
- Fluorescein angiography shows light bulb–like hyperfluorescence from the macroaneurysm
  - Alterations in the foveal circulation may be identified to explain decreased visual acuity
- Indocyanine green may be useful to identify the macroaneurysm when extensive intraretinal hemorrhage is present
- Ultrasound when diffuse vitreous hemorrhage prevents visualization of the retina or massive subretinal hemorrhage mimics choroidal melanoma
- Optical coherence tomography to identify macular edema

Differential Diagnosis

- Age-related macular degeneration with choroidal neovascularization • Diabetic retinopathy • Hypertensive retinopathy • Branch retinal vein occlusion • Coats disease • Capillary hemangioma • Choroidal melanoma (when massive subretinal hemorrhage present)

Treatment
- Observation when there is no macular edema or exudates in the fovea, because most macroaneurysms spontaneously resolve
- Argon laser photocoagulation in a grid pattern around the aneurysm or as light burns directly to the macroaneurysm to speed macular edema and exudate reabsorption
  - Caution should be used when directly treating macroaneurysms because they may rupture
- Pars plana vitrectomy for non-clearing vitreous hemorrhage
- Submacular surgery to remove non-clearing, thick submacular hemorrhage may be beneficial, but its utility is unproven
- Nd : YAG laser to release preretinal hemorrhage encapsulated by the internal limiting membrane or epiretinal membrane into the vitreous for more rapid clearance
- Intravitreal steroids for persistent macular edema

Prognosis
- **Visual prognosis may be fauorable if:**
  - there is no alteration of the foveal circulation • exudate does not accumulate in the fovea • macular edema resolves
- Direct laser photocoagulation may lead to rupture of the macroaneurysm or alteration of foveal circulation
- The presence of thick submacular hemorrhage, extensive exudate, or persistent macular edema portends a poor prognosis

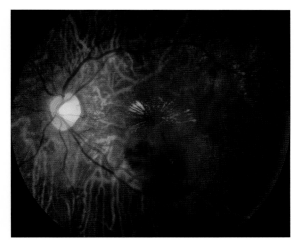

Fig. 3.35 An arterial macroaneurysm is present along the inferior temporal arcade. Subretinal hemorrhage surrounds the aneurysm with stellate exudate of the fovea.

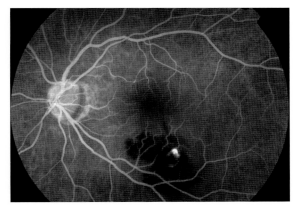

Fig. 3.36 Fluorescein angiogram of the eye in Figure 3.35 with light bulb-like hyperfluorescence.

Purtscher's Retinopathy

Key Facts

- Retinal changes occurring from compression injury to chest or head
- Complement activation and leukoembolization may induce vaso-occlusion and retinal ischemia
- Monocular or binocular
- May occur in any age group
- Ocular findings typically located around optic nerve

Clinical Findings

- Cotton wool spots
- Intraretinal hemorrhage
- Retinal edema
- Optic atrophy (chronic)

Ancillary Testing

- Fluorescein angiography to evaluate extent of arteriolar obstruction and non-perfusion
- Neurosurgical or general surgery consultation should be obtained if there is head or thoracoabdominal injury

Differential Diagnosis

- Hypertensive retinopathy
- Fat embolism from long bone fractures or crush injuries
- Pancreatitis (Purtscher-like retinopathy)
- Shaken baby syndrome
- Terson syndrome

Treatment

- Observation

Prognosis

- Permanent visual loss may occur from arteriolar obstruction and retinal infraction

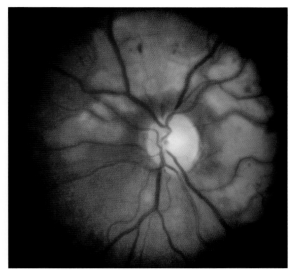

Fig. 3.37 Retinal edema, whitening, and cotton wool spots in an eye with Purtscher retinopathy.

Terson Syndrome

Key Facts

- Intraocular hemorrhage associated with acute intracranial hemorrhage
- Occurs in up to 20% of patients with acute intracranial bleeding
- Subarachnoid hemorrhage is the most common type
- Exact etiology of the intraocular hemorrhages is unknown but probably related to a rapid rise in intracranial pressure causing an acute rise in intraocular venous pressure that ruptures retinal or peripapillary vessels
- Usually bilateral
- Can affect all age groups but mainly occurs in the 30- to 50-year-old age group
- No sexual or racial predilection

Clinical Findings

- Intraretinal hemorrhage
- Subretinal hemorrhage
- Subhyaloid hemorrhage
- Vitreous hemorrhage

Ancillary Testing

- Neurosurgical consultation

Differential Diagnosis

- Proliferative diabetic retinopathy
- Shaken baby syndrome
- Blood dyscrasia
- Valsalva retinopathy
- Retinal tear
- Venous occlusive disease
- Arterial macroaneurysm
- Purtscher retinopathy

Treatment

- Observation because the retinal or vitreous hemorrhage usually spontaneously clears
- Pars plana vitrectomy when vitreous or subhyaloid hemorrhage is non-clearing
  - In the presence of a subhyaloid hemorrhage, the posterior hyaloid will need to be entered and peeled to access the blood

Prognosis

- Visual acuity usually not affected

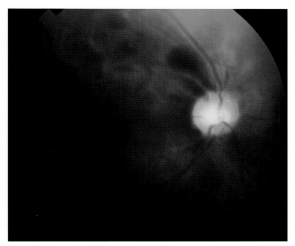

Fig. 3.38 Intraretinal hemorrhage from Terson syndrome in a patient who suffered a ruptured intracranial aneurysm and subarachnoid hemorrhage.

HIV Retinopathy

Key Facts

- Retinal findings due to HIV infection
- Rare finding because patients are asymptomatic
- Bilateral

Clinical Findings

- Cotton wool spots
- Retinal hemorrhages
- Microaneurysms

Ancillary Testing

- Evaluation for HIV

Differential Diagnosis

- Diabetic retinopathy
- Hypertensive retinopathy
- Venous occlusive disease
- Purtscher retinopathy
- Radiation retinopathy

Treatment

- Treat underlying HIV

Prognosis

- Cotton wool spots resolve within 6 weeks without visual sequelae

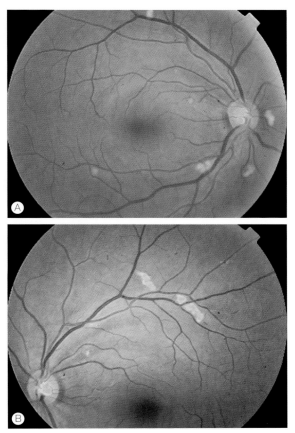

Fig. 3.39 Cotton wool spots in the (**A**) right and (**B**) left eye of this 31-year-old man. Testing showed that he was HIV-positive.

Hematologic Disorders

Key Facts

- Caused by changes in blood composition that alter blood flow characteristics
- Occurs with severe anemia, leukemia, thrombocytopenia, and macroglobulinemia
- Men and women equally affected
- No racial predilection

Clinical Findings

- Intraretinal or flame-shaped hemorrhage with or without white centers
- Subhyaloid hemorrhage
- Cotton wool spots
- Optic disc swelling
- Venous dilation
- Serous retinal detachment

Ancillary Testing

- Measure blood pressure to evaluate for hypertension
- **Obtain complete blood count to evaluate for abnormalities**

Differential Diagnosis

- Hypertensive retinopathy
- Diabetic retinopathy
- Terson syndrome

Treatment

- Treat the underlying hematologic disorder

Prognosis

- Vision rarely affected

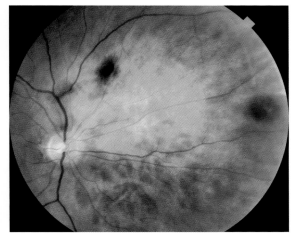

Fig. 3.40 Diffuse blot hemorrhages in a patient with acute myelogenous leukemia.

Section 4

Pediatric

Retinopathy of Prematurity

Key Facts

- Abnormal proliferation of developing retinal blood vessels at junction of vascularized and avascular retina in premature infants • Leading cause of childhood blindness in the USA • Clinical findings based on stage, zone, and presence or absence of plus disease • Greatest risk factors for developing retinopathy of prematurity (ROP) include lower birth weight and lower gestational age • In infants <1251 g, 65.8% showed ROP, with 6% reaching threshold disease in the Cryotherapy for Retinopathy of Prematurity (CRYO-ROP) trial

Clinical Findings

- Immature retina when vessels fade before reaching the ora serrata
- Staging of severity of disease
  - Stage 1: demarcation line • Stage 2: elevated, non-vascularized ridge • Stage 3: elevated, vascular ridge • Stage 4: partial retinal detachment that either spares (stage 4a) or involves (stage 4b) the fovea • Stage 5: total retinal detachment
- **Zone:** location of disease
  - Zone 1: circle centered on the optic nerve with the radius twice the distance from the disc to the fovea • Zone 2: extension of the circle centered on the optic nerve extending out to the nasal ora serrata • Zone 3: residual temporal retina left from the creation of zone 2
- **Plus disease:** presence of dilated and/or tortuous vessels at optic nerve head
- Temporal macular dragging • Macular fold • Vitreous hemorrhage • Cataract • Refractive errors • Strabismus • Amblyopia

Ancillary Testing

- Ultrasound if view to retina is poor

Differential Diagnosis

- Familial exudative vitreoretinopathy • Persistent hyperplastic primary vitreous (persistent fetal vasculature syndrome) • Retinoblastoma • Norrie disease • Incontinentia pigmenti

Treatment

- Screening for ROP should be performed in all infants <1500 g, of gestational age <28 weeks, or of 1500–2000 g birth weight believed to be at high risk • Examinations should take place 4–6 weeks after birth or 31–33 weeks postconception • Initiation of treatment by the CRYO-ROP study occurs when threshold disease (defined as five contiguous or eight total clock hours of stage 3, zone 1 or 2 with plus disease) is present • The Early Treatment for Retinopathy of Prematurity (ET-ROP) trial recommends treatment at zone 1 any stage with plus disease, zone 1 stage 3 with or without plus disease, or zone 2 stage 2 or 3 with plus disease • Laser photocoagulation to the area of avascular retina between the vascularized ridge and ora serrata is the current standard of care • Retinal detachments in stage 4 and 5 ROP are treated with scleral buckle or pars plana vitrectomy

Prognosis

- CRYO-ROP showed a 50% reduction of adverse structural outcomes and severe visual loss with early detection and treatment • 44.4% of treated eyes in CRYO-ROP had visual acuity of 20/200 or worse at 10 years • ET-ROP showed a reduction in unfavorable visual acuity outcomes by grating methods compared with CRYO-ROP at 9 months after treatment • 0.5% of patients with ROP will require vitrectomy or scleral buckle • Visual prognosis in eyes with stage 4 or 5 ROP is very poor

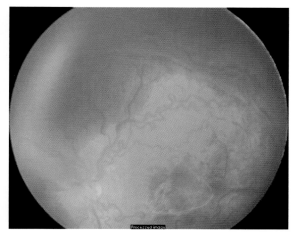

Fig. 4.1 Threshold ROP in this premature infant with stage 3 disease bordering zone 1 and zone 2 and the presence of plus disease. (Courtesy of Audina Berrocal, MD.)

Familial Exudative Vitreoretinopathy

Key Facts
- Disorder resembling retinopathy of prematurity but lacking history of premature birth
- Autosomal dominant with incomplete penetrance
- Bilateral disorder, often with asymmetric presentation
- Rate of progression of disease variable among affected patients
- Affects all age groups but more severe in patients <30 years
- About 50% of all patients are asymptomatic

Clinical Findings
- Avascular peripheral retina most prominent temporally but may involve entire peripheral retina
- Peripheral vascular sheathing
- Straightening of retinal vessels as they approach zone between perfused and non-perfused retina
- Peripheral retinal neovascularization
- Peripheral retinal traction
- Temporal macular dragging
- Macular fold
- Retinal exudates
- Intraretinal and subretinal hemorrhage
- Rhegmatogenous retinal detachment
- Non-rhegmatogenous retinal detachment (exudative or tractional)
- Strabismus (presentation in infants)
- Leukocoria (presentation in infants)

Ancillary Testing
- Retinal examination of all family members
- Fluorescein angiography will show peripheral avascular retina
  - Neovascularization may be seen at junction of perfused and non-perfused retina and will show active leakage

Differential Diagnosis
- Retinopathy of prematurity
- Coats disease
- Sickle cell
- Eales disease
- Toxocara
- Incontinentia pigmenti

Treatment
- Observation
- Laser photocoagulation to peripheral avascular retina
- Pars plana vitrectomy and/or scleral buckle for retinal detachment

Prognosis
- Vision loss and progression of disease more common within first three decades, with most eyes in this group achieving visual acuity of 20/200 or less
- Disease progression in adults is slower, affects vision less severely than in children, and tends to be more asymmetric
- Severe disease may lead to neovascular glaucoma and phthisis

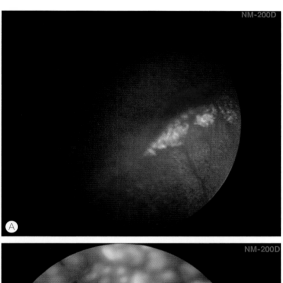

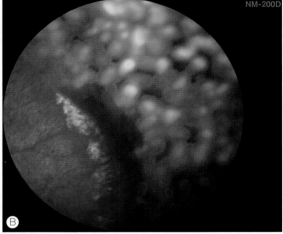

Fig. 4.2 A 7-week-old term baby was diagnosed with a total retinal detachment in the left eye and peripheral vascular changes in the right eye (**A**). The infant was diagnosed with familial exudative vitreoretinopathy. Peripheral laser to avascular retina was performed given the active neovascular process (**B**). (Courtesy of Dal Chun, MD.)

Persistent Fetal Vasculature

Key Facts

- Formerly known as persistent hyperplastic primary vitreous • Failure of primary vitreous and hyaloid vasculature to regress, with eventual contraction and opacification • Etiology unknown • Anterior and posterior forms exist • Unilateral in 90% of cases • Varying degrees of severity • No sexual predilection • No systemic abnormalities reported • Sporadic inheritance in vast majority of cases • Leukocoria identified soon after birth • Retinoblastoma must be excluded

Clinical Findings

- Retrolental, white fibrous membrane • Microphthalmia • Shallow anterior chamber • Elongated ciliary processes • Cataract • Esotropia • Angle closure glaucoma • Dilated iris vessels • Persistent hyaloid artery • Vitreous hemorrhage
- Stalk of tissue from optic disc toward the retrolental region that may run along a retinal fold
  - The stalk may fan out toward the anterior retina
- Retinal detachment

Ancillary Testing

- CT scan of orbit to evaluate for the presence of calcification, which is present in retinoblastoma but absent in persistent fetal vasculature • B-scan ultrasonography to evaluate for retinal detachment when cataract limits the view to the retina

Differential Diagnosis

- Congenital cataract • Retinoblastoma • Coats disease • Familial exudative vitreoretinopathy • Toxocariasis • Uveitis • Norrie disease • Incontinentia pigmenti

Treatment

- Observation in mild cases • Pars plana lensectomy and vitrectomy to remove the retrolental fibrovascular membrane to prevent angle closure glaucoma, followed by aggressive amblyopia therapy

Prognosis

- Natural course of disease leads to blindness in advanced cases • Surgery effective in restoring vision in only a small percentage of eyes • Because the disease is almost always unilateral, amblyopia is a significant cause of poor vision in affected eyes

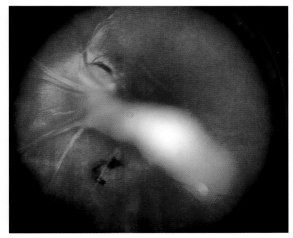

Fig. 4.3 A fibrovascular stalk extends from the optic nerve in persistent fetal vasculature.

Shaken Baby Syndrome

Key Facts

- Retinal findings that occur following violent shaking of an infant
- Clinical findings are usually bilateral

Clinical Findings

- Diffuse intraretinal hemorrhage
- Subretinal hemorrhage
- Vitreous or subhyaloid hemorrhage
- Optic disc swelling
- Cotton wool spots
- Venous engorgement
- Chorioretinal atrophy (chronic)

Ancillary Testing

- Ultrasound when vitreous hemorrhage present
- Consultation with a pediatrician to evaluate for systemic findings of child abuse including long bone fractures and intracranial hemorrhage
- Complete blood count to evaluate for blood dyscrasias

Differential Diagnosis

- Leukemia
- Purtscher's retinopathy
- Terson syndrome
- Central retinal vein occlusion
- Birth trauma

Treatment

- Observation
- Vitreous hemorrhage that occludes visual axis and fails to rapidly clear may require pars plana vitrectomy to prevent amblyopia

Prognosis

- Poor visual prognosis when there is extensive chorioretinal atrophy, deprivation amblyopia, or brain injury

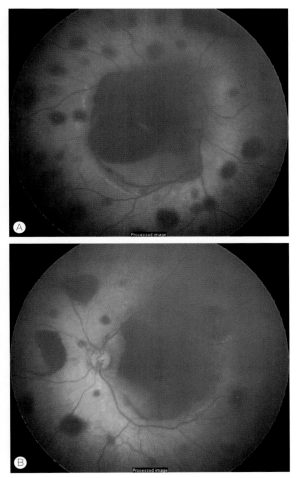

Fig. 4.4 Intraretinal (**A**) and panretinal (**B**) hemorrhage in shaken baby syndrome (Courtesy of Audina Berrocal, MD).

Section 5

Trauma

Commotio Retina

Key Facts
- Concussive injury to retina from blunt trauma
- Occurs within a few hours of injury
- Most common in young males

Clinical Findings
- Retinal whitening in macula and/or peripheral retina
- Retinal hemorrhage
- Vitreous hemorrhage
- Choroidal rupture
- Macular hole
- Chronic foveal retinal pigment epithelium (RPE) alterations
- Retinal dialysis
- Avulsion of vitreous base

Ancillary Testing
- Clinical examination only

Differential Diagnosis
- White without pressure
- Retinal detachment

Treatment
- Observation

Prognosis
- Vision usually recovers within 3–4 weeks
- Chronic visual decline is due to macular hole formation or RPE changes at fovea

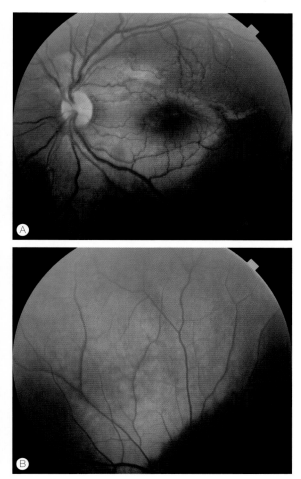

Fig. 5.1 Commotio retina after blunt trauma. The retinal whitening is focused in the macula (**A**) and extends out to the peripheral retina (**B**).

Light Toxicity

Key Facts

- Light-induced retinal damage
- Ophthalmic instruments (endoillumination during vitrectomy or microscope light during anterior segment surgery), sun gazing, arc welding, and industrial lasers are common causes
- Patients may be asymptomatic, complain of decreased vision, or notice scotomas

Clinical Findings

- May be barely visible
- Yellow spot with retinal edema in acute injury
- Bilateral focal pigmentary changes (reddish or yellow foveal reflex) in solar retinopathy
- Pigmentary changes at or near fovea from healed lesions

Ancillary Testing

- Optical coherence tomography shows thinning of retina at fovea, with variable photoreceptor loss
- Window defect and staining occur on fluorescein angiography at area of scar tissue

Differential Diagnosis

- Age-related macular degeneration
- Pattern dystrophy

Treatment

- Observation

Prognosis

- Vision usually improves but full recovery depends on extent and location of damage
- Patients may experience a permanent central or paracentral scotoma

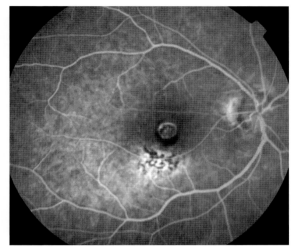

Fig. 5.2 Staining of scar in the macula from light toxicity that occurred during cataract surgery from the light source on an operating microscope.

Posterior Lens Dislocation

Key Facts

- Displacement of lens into vitreous cavity
- **Occurs secondary to:**
    - trauma • intraoperative rupture of posterior lens capsule • pseudoexfoliation
        - inherited familial disorders (Marfan syndrome, Weill–Marchesani syndrome)
        - metabolic disorders (sulfite oxidase deficiency, homocystinuria)
- Immediate decrease in visual acuity
- Trauma and surgical complications are monocular
- Pseudoexfoliation, familial and metabolic disorders are bilateral

Clinical Findings

- Lens (either entire lens or pieces of lens material from surgery) in vitreous cavity
- Intraocular inflammation
- Elevated IOP from phacolytic glaucoma
- Vitreous hemorrhage from trauma or surgery
- Iridodonesis

Ancillary Testing

- Ultrasound if view to the retina is poor
- Evaluation for metabolic or familial disorders in conjunction with primary care physician

Differential Diagnosis

- Based on the metabolic or familial cause of the lens dislocation

Treatment

- Observation if no intraocular inflammation or elevated IOP from the dislocated lens
- Pars plana vitrectomy with lensectomy should be performed immediately after complicated cataract surgery or traumatic displacement of the lens if elevated IOP cannot be controlled with maximal medical therapy
- Surgical placement of an appropriate intraocular lens implant during vitrectomy surgery
- If no lens implant is performed, aphakic correction with contact lens may be used

Prognosis

- Good visual prognosis

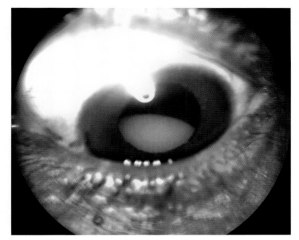

Fig. 5.3 A mature, white dislocated lens from previous trauma in the inferior vitreous cavity.

Intraocular Foreign Body

Key Facts

- Occurs when a high-velocity object penetrates the eye • Metallic intraocular foreign bodies (IOFBs) are the most common, with hammering metal on metal the most common setting • Patient history may be the most useful information in identifying the presence and material of a foreign body • Occurs primarily in 20- to 40-year-old men • Complete eye examination including visual acuity should be performed, while avoiding any further damage to the eye

Clinical Findings

- Conjunctival injection • Subconjunctival hemorrhage • Localized or diffuse hemorrhagic chemosis • Scleral or corneal laceration with uveal or vitreous prolapse, or occult with a self-sealing wound • IOP may be low, normal, or elevated • Hyphema • Vitreous hemorrhage • Intraocular inflammation • Cataract • Lens dislocation • Irregular pupil • Retinal detachment • Endophthalmitis • Metallosis

Ancillary Testing

- Ultrasound to evaluate for IOFBs, retinal detachment, and choroidal hemorrhage
  - if a cornea or scleral laceration present, pressure on the globe from an ultrasound probe may further injure the eye
- CT more accurately identifies the presence of a foreign body in the globe or orbit than ultrasound or x-ray and is the standard imaging technique
  - CT can identify both metallic and non-metallic IOFBs but may miss wooden objects
  - CT is less accurate than ultrasound in identifying retinal detachment and choroidal hemorrhage
- Plain film x-ray may be used in the absence of CT but is far less accurate in localizing foreign bodies
- MRI should be avoided in the case of a suspected metallic IOFB
- Electroretinogram (ERG) to evaluate for the presence of metallic retinal toxicity from a chronic IOFB

Differential Diagnosis

- Blunt trauma
- Corneal or scleral laceration without IOFB
- Conjunctival laceration

Treatment

- Primary closure of cornea or scleral wounds and removal of IOFB with cultures of the foreign body should be done within 24 h of acute injury when possible
- Removal of IOFB internally via pars plana approach with intraocular forceps and intraocular rare earth magnet or externally by magnet
  - Pars plana approach is most often used given advances in intraocular surgery
  - External magnets may be used for small metallic IOFBs that that are not incarcerated, are clearly visualized, and whose removal will not injure the retina or lens
- Repair of retinal detachment by pars plana vitrectomy or scleral buckle
- Prophylactic systemic antibiotics (vancomycin with a third-generation cephalosporin) for 1–3 days, followed by an oral antibiotic for endophthalmitis prophylaxis

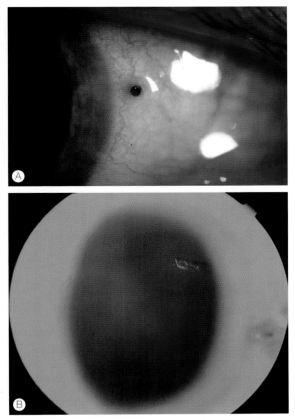

Fig. 5.4 A metallic IOFB impaled in the sclera (**A**) and penetrating the vitreous cavity (**B**) through the pars plana is visible at the slit lamp. The piece of metal was removed at the slit lamp without complication.

- Intravitreal vancomycin (1 mg/0.1 mL) and ceftazidime (2.25 mg/0.1 mL) when endophthalmitis highly suspicious or clinically present
- With chronic inert IOFBs, close observation with serial ERG is adequate
    - removal of the IOFB is required if there is any decline in ERG, vision, or ocular status

Prognosis

- **Visual outcome depends on:**
    - presenting visual acuity
    - presence of afferent pupillary defect
    - endophthalmitis
    - extent of tissue loss at time of injury
    - formation of proliferative vitreoretinopathy
    - damage to macula either directly from the IOFB or indirectly from blunt trauma
- The risk of endophthalmitis ranges from 6–13%, depending on the study; however, rates of endophthalmitis with organic matter may be as high as 30%, with most cases due to *Bacillus* species

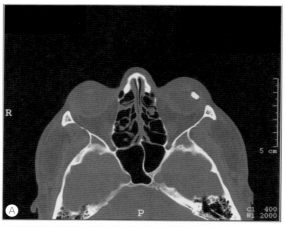

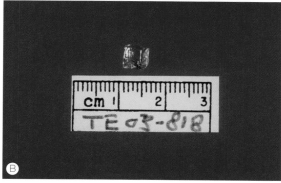

Fig. 5.5 CT scan (**A**) of a glass IOFB from a sidecar window (**B**) removed from the left vitreous cavity following a motor vehicle accident.

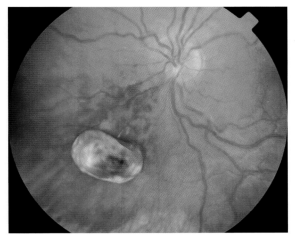

Fig. 5.6 An encapsulated inert IOFB in the eye of a teenaged boy; it had been observed for 6 years without complication.

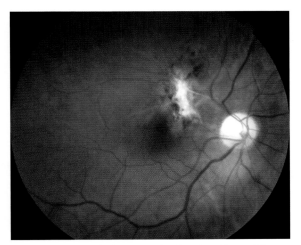

Fig. 5.7 A chorioretinal scar marks the site of impact from a metallic foreign body that was removed during pars plana vitrectomy. The IOFB severed the superior temporal retinal artery and vein, inducing the retinal hemorrhages noted distal to the scar. The vision remains counting fingers.

Choroidal Rupture

Key Facts

- Occurs from blunt trauma that compresses the globe, inducing a tearing or disruption of the choroid, choriocapillaris, Bruch's membrane, and retinal pigment epithelium (RPE)
- Most choroidal ruptures occur in the posterior retina from indirect forces induced by the trauma

Clinical Findings

- Yellow-white line that is crescent-shaped or concentric with optic nerve
- Choroidal ruptures that are more chronic will have pigmentation at the edges from RPE migration
- Subretinal hemorrhage
- Vitreous hemorrhage
- Commotio retina
- Hyphema
- Lens subluxation
- Iris sphincter tears
- Angle recession
- Retinal tear
- Retinal dialysis
- Choroidal neovascularization (CNV) adjacent to or along choroidal rupture (late finding)

Ancillary tests

- Fluorescein angiography to evaluate for presence of CNV—the edge of the choroidal rupture stains during the angiogram
- Visual field to evaluate for scotomas or enlarged blind spots

Differential Diagnosis

- CNV
- Lacquer cracks from myopia
- Angioid streaks
- Retinal arterial macroaneurysm
- Valsalva retinopathy
- Penetrating trauma with an intraocular foreign body

Treatment

- Observation
- CNV may be treated with intravitreal anti–vascular endothelial growth factor injections
  - currently, no studies or publications support this method of treatment

Prognosis

- Visual outcome varies and depends on late pigmentary changes and atrophy in the macula, location of rupture through the fovea, and formation of CNV

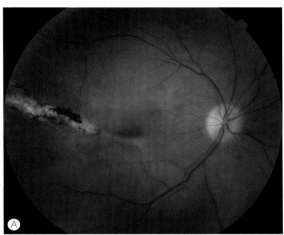

Fig. 5.8 (**A**) A chronic choroidal rupture traversing through the fovea. The rupture is chronic given the presence of pigment along the rupture site. A wing-shaped area of fibrosis in the fovea represents CNV. (**B**) Fluorescein angiogram shows that the CNV stains and is inactive.

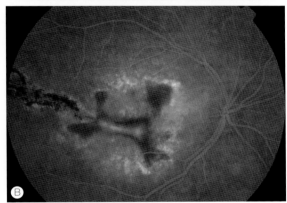

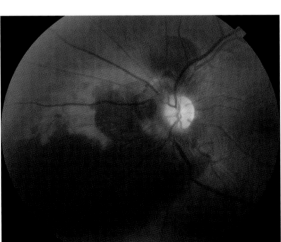

Fig. 5.9 Subretinal hemorrhage surrounding the optic nerve from severe blunt trauma to the eye.

Section 6

Tumors

Choroidal Nevus

Key Facts

- Benign tumor of the choroid • Most common primary intraocular tumor • No sexual predilection • Most are congenital but do not become pigmented until after childhood • Become more clinically evident with increasing age • More common in persons with lightly pigmented skin • Typically unilateral • Bilateral, multiple nevi rarely occur in neurofibromatosis type 1 and systemic carcinoma

Clinical Findings

- Gray-brown choroidal lesion with feathered edges • Occasionally amelanotic • Homogenous surface but drusen or pigmentary changes may be present • Basal diameter of 5–10 mm • Elevation of ≤1 mm is common but thickness of 3 mm or more may occur • Serous detachment overlying nevus • Choroidal neovascularization (CNV) rarely occurs and does not imply malignant transformation

Ancillary Testing

- Baseline photograph for documentation • Ultrasound to measure lesion height in nevi suspicious for being malignant choroidal melanoma • Choroidal nevi are hypofluorescent on fluorescein angiography, without evidence of intralesional circulation (as seen in a malignant choroidal melanoma) • Nevi are non-fluorescent on indocyanine green angiography • Fine needle aspiration in suspicious choroidal nevi • Because the vast majority of choroidal nevi are benign, systemic evaluation is unnecessary

Differential Diagnosis

- Choroidal melanoma • Congenital hypertrophy of the retinal pigment epithelium (CHRPE) • Metastatic carcinoma • Hyperplasia of the RPE • Choroidal osteoma • Subretinal or suprachoroidal hemorrhage

Treatment

- Observation with follow-up based on level of suspicion of malignancy
  - Examination is performed every 1–2 years for nevi without suspicion for malignant potential—most lesions change very little over time • Lesions suspicious for choroidal melanoma should be followed more closely, with dilated examinations and ultrasound measurement of lesion height every 1–3 months
- Leaking nevi with serous detachments may be treated with observation, focal laser to the point of leakage, or barrier laser around the nevus to prevent leakage into the fovea
  - Many leaking nevi will spontaneously cease, so a trial of observation is recommended • Focal laser may result in rupture of Bruch's membrane • Laser is also limited when nevi are present at or near the fovea
- Treatment of CNV historically consists of focal laser
  - Intravitreal anti–vascular endothelial growth factor may be considered

Prognosis

- Malignant transformation is rare, occurring in about 1 in 8000

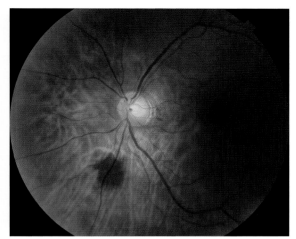

Fig. 6.1 Flat choroidal nevus located inferior to the optic disc.

Melanocytoma of the Optic Nerve

Key Facts

- Benign pigmented tumor situated on optic disc
- Variant of choroidal nevus
- No sexual predilection
- Occurs equally in caucasians and African Americans

Clinical Findings

- Dark brown-black lesion situated on optic disc
- Indistinct, feathery margins due to the presence of the nerve fiber layer
- Lesions are flat or minimally elevated
- Slow growth may occur
- Visual field defect

Ancillary Testing

- Photographic documentation of lesion to monitor for growth
- The lesion is hypofluorescent on fluorescein angiography, which differentiates melanocytoma from malignant melanoma
- Visual field test to evaluate for defects secondary to compression of optic disc

Differential Diagnosis

- Choroidal melanoma
- Choroidal nevus

Treatment

- Observation

Prognosis

- Vast majority of lesions are benign and do not lead to visual impairment

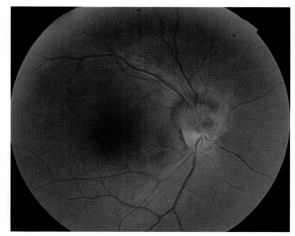
Fig. 6.2 Melanocytoma of the optic nerve.

Congenital Hypertrophy of the Retinal Pigment Epithelium

Key Facts
- Uncommon congenital lesion
- Men and women equally affected
- All racial groups equally affected
- Lesions asymptomatic and detected on routine ophthalmic examination
- **Occurs in one of three forms:**
  1. single monocular lesion (common) 2. multifocal unilateral lesion (common)
     3. multifocal bilateral bear track lesions (rare with risk of familial adenomatous polyposis of the colon)
- Familial adenomatous polyposis occurs in about 1 in 100 000 people

Clinical Findings
- Round, darkly pigmented lesion
- Well-demarcated, sharp borders
- Hypopigmented halo may surround lesion
- Hypopigmented lacunae occur as lesion ages

Ancillary Testing
- Rarely required—diagnosis based primarily on clinical examination
- Photographic documentation
- On fluorescein angiography, the lesion is hypofluorescent without leaking throughout the angiogram
  - Lacunar areas demonstrate window defect

Differential Diagnosis
- Choroidal nevus
- Choroidal melanoma
- Melanocytoma
- Reactive hyperplasia of retinal pigment epithelium (RPE)
- Subretinal blood
- Adenoma or adenocarcinoma of RPE
- Combined hamartoma of retina and RPE
- Toxoplasmosis scar

Treatment
- Observation
- If lesions are atypical, multifocal, and bilateral, patients should be referred for colonoscopy given the risk of colon cancer from familial adenomatous polyposis

Prognosis
- Lesions usually stable and require observation every year or two
- Malignant transformation rare
- Vision not affected

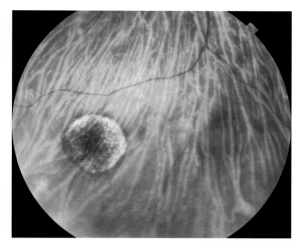

Fig. 6.3 Congenital hypertrophy of the retinal pigment epithelium.

Retinoblastoma

Key Facts

- Most common intraocular malignancy in childhood
- No sexual or racial predilection
- Occurs in 1 in 15 000 live births
- Caused by the inactivation of both alleles of the retinoblastoma gene located on the long arm of chromosome 13
- 6% of newly diagnosed cases are familial, 94% sporadic
- Unilateral cases are the most common, and tumors in these eyes are typically unifocal
  - bilateral cases tend to have multifocal disease
- Diagnosed at an average age of 12 months in unilateral cases and 24 months in bilateral cases
- Invades the optic nerve and sclera, extends into the brain, and has the ability to metastasize
- Trilateral retinoblastoma is a combination of bilateral retinoblastoma and pinealoblastoma

Clinical Findings

- Leukocoria
- Exotropia or esotropia
- White dome-shaped mass that is endophytic (grows from the retina into the vitreous cavity), exophytic (grows from the retina into the subretinal space), or diffusely infiltrating (rare)
- Dilated and tortuous retinal arteries and veins feeding the tumor
- Vitreous seeds
- Iris nodules
- Clear lens
- Pseudohypopyon
- Exudative retinal detachment
- Iris neovascularization
- Iris heterochromia
- Hyphema
- Periocular inflammation from a necrotic retinoblastoma
- Pinealoblastoma

Ancillary Testing

- Fluorescein angiography is difficult to obtain in infants
  - Fine capillaries are identified on the surface of the tumor that hyperfluoresce during the angiogram
- The tumor on B scan shows increased reflectivity due to the presence of calcium in the tumor, with shadowing behind the lesion
  - When the gain is reduced, the reflectivity of the calcified tumor persists • High reflective spikes in the tumor occur on A-scan ultrasonography
- On MRI, the tumor is moderately hyperintense on T_1-weighted images and hypointense on T_2-weighted images
  - Extraocular tumor extension and the presence of pinealoblastoma may be evaluated
- On CT, retinoblastoma has multiple foci of calcification within the tumor
  - Calcification may be seen in other disorders (e.g. Coats disease), therefore this finding is not pathognomonic for retinoblastoma • Extraocular extension and pinealoblastoma may be detected • To avoid radiation exposure from CT in young children, MRI is recommended for imaging of the orbits and brain
- Examination under anesthesia to ensure a thorough retinal examination of both eyes to rule out peripheral tumor that may be missed on examination in the office
- Genetic counseling, especially in familial or bilateral cases
- Complete blood count

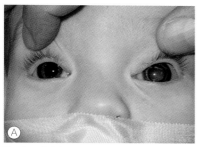
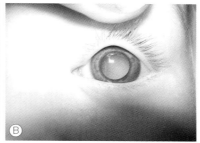

Fig. 6.4 (**A**) External photograph showing leukocoria of the left eye from retinoblastoma. (**B**) A close-up of the affected eye shows a retinal detachment (Courtesy of Gary L. Rogers, MD).

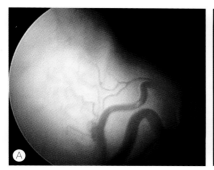
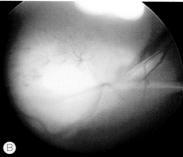

Fig. 6.5 (**A**) An exophytic retinoblastoma with a dilated vein and artery. (**B**) An associated exudative retinal detachment is present.

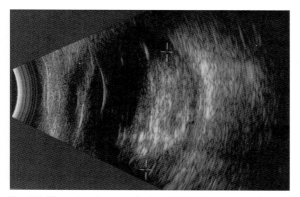

Fig. 6.6 B-mode ultrasound of the retinoblastoma in Fig. 6.5, showing areas of increased reflectivity within the tumor and acoustic shadowing into the orbit.

Retinoblastoma (Continued)

Differential Diagnosis

- Coats disease
- Congenital cataract
- Retinopathy of prematurity
- Coloboma
- Toxocariasis
- Persistent fetal vasculature
- Astrocytic hamartoma
- Combined hamartoma
- Vitreous hemorrhage
- Rhegmatogenous retinal detachment
- Myelinated nerve fiber layer
- Uveitis

Treatment

- Enucleation is recommended for all unilateral tumors that are extensive with poor visual prognosis or in extensive bilateral disease when visual prognosis is poor
  - A long section of the optic nerve must be obtained, because the optic nerve is the main route of extension of retinoblastoma cells into the central nervous system
- Chemotherapy is used for bilateral disease or extraocular extension and as initial therapy in unilateral disease when the eye is felt to be salvageable
  - Carboplatin, etoposide, and vincristine are used in six cycles spaced 3–4 weeks apart—most regression occurs within the first two cycles • Any residual tumor is then treated with photocoagulation, cryotherapy, or radiation plaque
    - If vitreous seeds persist, external beam irradiation is used
- External beam irradiation may be used to treat the second eye after the eye with the more advanced tumor has been enucleated
  - Side effects include the formation of tumors (sarcoma in the field of irradiation, leukemia, and lymphoma)
- Cryotherapy is useful for small peripheral tumors without vitreous seeding
  - The treatment is repeated every 2–4 weeks until the tumor has regressed
- Argon laser photocoagulation is applied around small tumors with a basal diameter of 7 mm and a maximum height of 2–3 mm that are located outside the macula
  - The tumors are encircled with laser every 3–4 weeks to cut off the vascular supply feeding the retinoblastoma • Treatment is repeated until an atrophic scar is present • Laser is not directed at the tumor, to prevent rupture and release of tumor cells
- Transpupillary thermotherapy allows direct treatment to the tumor with a 2- to 3-mm spot size for 60 s, with overlapping treatments, to create a mild whitening of the tumor
  - Treatment is repeated every 2–4 weeks until the tumor has regressed
- Scleral plaque brachytherapy is used as a primary or secondary treatment for unilateral or bilateral tumors
  - Most tumors show rapid regression.

Prognosis

- Death occurs within 2–4 years in untreated disease
- Metastatic disease or intracranial retinoblastoma ultimately leads to death despite chemotherapy
- 45% of eyes treated with eye-sparing therapy develop recurrent tumors
- Secondary malignancy often occurs in survivors of the disease with a germinal mutation
- Poor prognosis for life when trilateral retinoblastoma is present (bilateral retinoblastoma and pinealoblastoma)

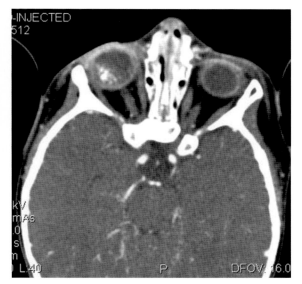

Fig. 6.7 CT scan of the orbits, with intraocular calcification in the right eye.

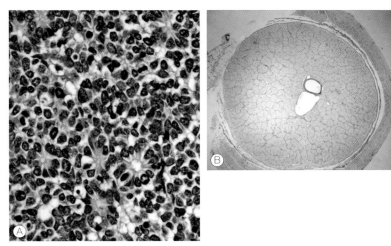

Fig. 6.8 (**A**) Histology section of the retinoblastoma from the enucleated eye of the patient in Fig. 6.5, showing Flexner–Wintersteiner rosettes. (**B**) There is no evidence of tumor in the section of the optic nerve.

Choroidal Melanoma

Key Facts

- Most common primary intraocular malignancy
- Primarily affects caucasians
- Incidence is about 1 in 2500 in caucasians
- Typically identified after age 30
- No inheritance pattern
- No sexual predilection but men may be slightly more affected
- Arises in ciliary body or choroid
- Unilateral and unifocal

Clinical Findings

- Dilated episcleral vessel
- Unilateral cataract
- Unilateral astigmatism
- Localized elevation of iris
- Elevated, dome-shaped, brown-pigmented lesion originating from choroid
- Orange pigment clumps on tumor surface
- Mushroom-shaped appearance if tumor breaks through Bruch's membrane
- Pigmentation may vary and the melanoma may be deemed an amelanotic melanoma
- Subretinal fluid may be bullous with shifting subretinal fluid
- Rare extension through sclera

Ancillary Testing

- Choroidal melanomas primarily diagnosed by clinical appearance
- Systemic work-up is required for evaluation of metastatic disease
  - This includes blood work evaluating liver function, chest x-ray and abdominal scan with CT or MRI to evaluate for liver metastases
- Color photographs of tumor for baseline documentation
- Transillumination casts a shadow from the pigmented melanoma that also allows for measurement of the base of the lesion in preparation for treatment
- Fluorescein angiography shows early hypofluorescence with filling of intralesional arterioles, with immediate leakage and staining following the arteriolar phase
- Indocyanine green angiography shows hypofluorescence throughout the entire study with well-delineated intralesional vessels
- A-scan ultrasound records a high initial spike with moderate to low internal reflectivity
- B-scan ultrasound images a dome- or mushroom-shaped lesion that is sonolucent
  - The height of the lesion is measured with B-mode ultrasound
  - Choroidal melanomas are generally >2 mm thick, with a minimum base of 7 mm
- Fine needle aspiration through a limbal approach in large ciliary body melanomas or via pars plana approach

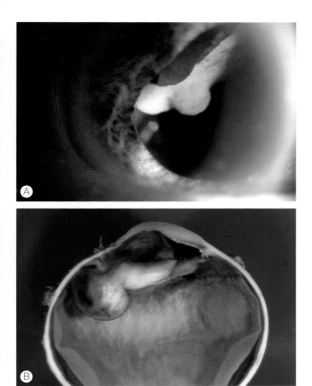

Fig. 6.9 (**A**) A ciliary body melanoma in an 80-year-old woman, with extension into the iris and anterior chamber. (**B**) The eye was enucleated, with the gross section of the eye present.

Differential Diagnosis

- Choroidal nevus
- Rhegmatogenous retinal detachment
- Metastatic tumor
- Congenital hypertrophy of the retinal pigment epithelium (CHRPE)
- Lymphoma
- Exudative age-related macular degeneration in the form of a submacular hemorrhage or peripheral choroidal neovascularization
- Limited suprachoroidal hemorrhage
- Melanocytoma
- Choroidal osteoma
- Choroidal hemangioma
- Leiomyoma
- Combined hamartoma of the retina and RPE
- Adenoma or adenocarcinoma
- Medulloepithelioma
- Nodular posterior scleritis

Treatment

- Observation at regular intervals if lesions are <2 mm in height and show no evidence of progressive growth
  - This is most appropriate when attempting to differentiate between a melanoma and a nevus
  - Observation of an obvious melanoma is not advised unless the patient is unable to undergo treatment
- Enucleation is the oldest method of treatment and is used in eyes that are blind and painful, that have very large tumors, or when tumor invades the optic nerve
  - Pre-enucleation radiation may be used when extrascleral extension of tumor is present
- Radioactive plaque brachytherapy emitting iodine-125 is commonly used for tumors <8 mm in height and 15 mm in basal diameter located ≥3 mm from the optic disc and fovea
  - The plaque is sutured to the sclera at the location of the base of the tumor in the operating room and remains on the eye for ≤7 days
- Proton beam irradiation is used for similar-sized tumors as with plaque radiation and is administered over 4–7 days
- Gamma knife irradiation is administered in one sitting and applies radiation from multiple angles to the tumor as mapped out on MRI obtained before treatment
- Transpupillary thermotherapy for lesions that are <4 mm high
- Argon laser photocoagulation
- Surgical resection

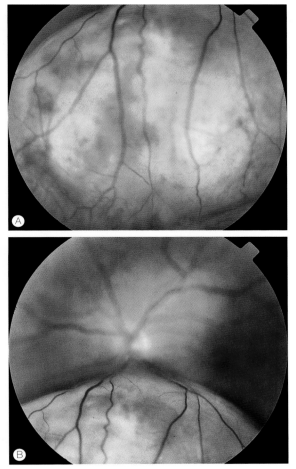

Fig. 6.10 A choroidal melanoma in the inferior retina, abutting the optic disc.

Prognosis

- At 10 years, there is a 34% risk of metastasis
- **Factors increasing the risk of metastasis include:**
    - older age • extrascleral extension • larger tumor size • location in ciliary body
- The Collaborative Ocular Melanoma Study showed no difference in mortality from metastatic disease from medium-sized choroidal melanoma in patients treated with enucleation versus plaque radiation
- Local tumor recurrence occurs in ≤10% of eyes treated with plaque radiation and ≤5% of eyes treated with external beam irradiation
- The natural history of untreated disease is not well documented
- Visual acuity after treatment depends on location of tumor with regard to optic nerve and macula

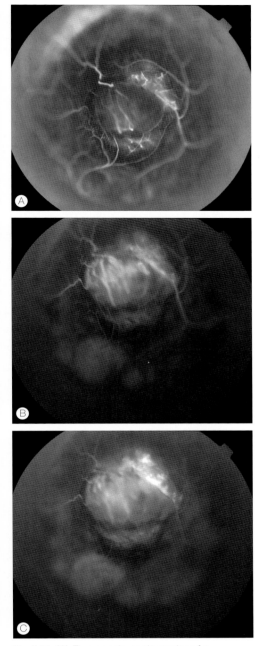

Fig. 6.11 (**A**) Fluorescein angiography of a choroidal melanoma shows early hypofluorescence with filling of the intralesional arterioles at 37 s. At (**B**) 2 min and (**C**) 5 min of the angiogram, there is progressive mild leakage.

Choroidal Hemangioma

Key Facts

- Rare, benign, vascular tumor of the choroid • Congenital • No racial or sexual predilection • Etiology unknown • Incidence unknown • No inheritance pattern • Symptoms occur in second to fourth decades • Usually unilateral • Occurs as an isolated, well-circumscribed tumor or as a diffuse tumor in Sturge–Weber syndrome (encephalofacial cavernous hemangiomatosis) • Diffuse choroidal hemangiomas are classified as part of Sturge–Weber syndrome when associated with leptomeningeal hemangiomas and intracranial calcification of the cerebral cortex

Clinical Findings

- **Circumscribed choroidal hemangiomas:**
  - oval, red-orange elevated tumor in or around the macula • subretinal fluid • non-rhegmatogenous retinal detachment • degeneration of retinal pigment epithelium in chronic lesions • exudation rarely occurs • hyperopic shift
- **Diffuse choroidal hemangioma:**
  - ipsilateral facial hemangioma (port wine stain) • diffuse, ipsilateral deep red appearance of the choroid (tomato catsup fundus) in the macula • amblyopia • hyperopic refractive error • elevated IOP • abnormal angle structures • dilated episcleral and scleral vessels • optic nerve cupping secondary to elevated IOP (especially when upper lid involved with nevus flammeus) • thickening of the choroid centered on optic nerve • non-rhegmatogenous retinal detachment

Ancillary Testing

- Ultrasonography in a circumscribed choroidal hemangioma shows a solid tumor with high internal reflectivity on A scan
  - A serous retinal detachment may be present around or overlying the tumor
  - In a diffuse choroidal hemangioma, there is a thickened choroid with medium to high internal reflectivity and a retinal detachment when present
- Fluorescein in a circumscribed choroidal hemangioma rapidly fills the intralesional and choroidal vessels just before the arterial phase, followed by leakage throughout the remaining phases of the angiogram
  - In a diffuse choroidal hemangioma, there is leakage similar to that seen with a circumscribed choroidal hemangioma but in more diffuse fashion
- Indocyanine green (ICG) is similar to fluorescein angiography, with early delineation of the intralesional choroidal vasculature followed by leakage
  - Washout of the ICG dye occurs centrally in the last frames, with persistent fluorescence of the outer edges of the tumor
- No systemic work-up is required for circumscribed choroidal hemangiomas

Differential Diagnosis

- Choroidal melanoma • Posterior scleritis • Choroidal osteoma

Treatment

- Treatment is initiated only if the lesion is vision-threatening or there is a non-rhegmatogenous retinal detachment
  - Asymptomatic patients should be observed
- Grid laser photocoagulation to the surface of the tumor to treat subretinal fluid
- Transpupillary thermotherapy
- Photodynamic therapy with verteporfin
- Radiation with proton beam or brachytherapy

Prognosis

- In diffuse choroidal hemangiomas, external beam irradiation is effective in inducing complete resolution of subretinal fluid
- Poor prognosis with macular lesions or extensive retinal detachment

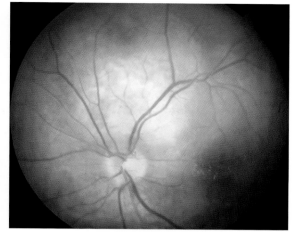

Fig. 6.12 A choroidal hemangioma superior to the optic nerve with exudate leaking into the fovea.

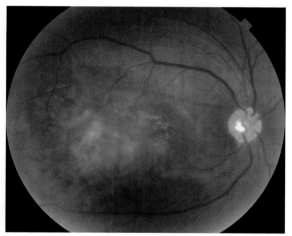

Fig. 6.13 A chronic choroidal hemangioma without active leakage in the macula, exhibiting metaplasia of the retinal pigment epithelium. The lesion has been present by history for 7 years and has induced a hyperopic shift.

Choroidal Metastases

Key Facts

- Neoplasm that hematogenously spreads to the choroid of the eye from an extraocular primary source • Most common intraocular malignancy • Most patients have a known primary extraocular lesion
- Affected eyes usually have a single monocular tumor
  - Multifocal monocular or bilateral choroidal metastases occur less commonly
- Tumors often asymptomatic and may not be identified until the patient is in the final stages of disease
- Breast cancer is the most common primary source in women
- Lung cancer is the most common primary source in men

Clinical Findings

- Round or oval elevated choroidal mass • Neoplasms are typically amelanotic with mottling of the retinal pigment epithelium • Non-rhegmatogenous retinal detachment

Ancillary Testing

- Color photograph
- Fluorescein angiography shows hypofluorescence in arterial phase given the absence of large intralesional vessels
  - Hyperfluorescence is visible in later frames of the angiogram, with occasional punctate hyperfluorescence
- Lesions hypofluorescent on indocyanine green throughout the entire study
- Metastatic lesions on ultrasound have a broad base compared with a choroidal malignant melanoma
  - Surrounding subretinal fluid from exudative retinal detachment may be present
- If no known previous malignancy, a full systemic evaluation is required in conjunction with a primary care physician and oncologist
  - With a known pre-existing malignancy, reconsultation with an oncologist to plan further systemic treatment is required

Differential Diagnosis

- Amelanotic choroidal melanoma • Amelanotic choroidal nevus • Choroidal hemangioma • Choroidal osteoma • Intraocular lymphoma • Posterior scleritis

Treatment

- Management should consider the patient's desire for further treatment and overall systemic health
- Radiation therapy is effective if vision is threatened with a tumor located in the macula or infiltrating the optic nerve
- Chemotherapy or hormonal therapy may be effective in tumors not affecting vision
- Observation

Prognosis

- Choroidal metastatic tumor growth is variable and may be rapid with associated exudative retinal detachment • Metastatic choroidal neoplasms represent poor prognosis for overall survival • Visual outcome depends on location and responsiveness to treatment

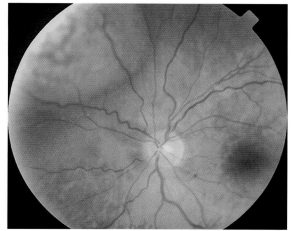
Fig. 6.14 Superior choroidal metastasis in a woman with known advanced metastatic breast cancer.

Intraocular Lymphoma

Key Facts

- Rare intraocular tumor • Usually B-cell, non-Hodgkin lymphomas • Bilateral involvement in ≤90% of patients • Most occur in immunocompetent persons in the sixth and seventh decades • Immunosuppressed patients can be affected at a younger age • No sexual or racial predilection • Associated with primary central nervous system (CNS) lymphoma in >50% of cases and systemic lymphoma in about 15% of cases • Isolated intraocular lymphoma occurs, but CNS involvement eventually occurs with extended follow-up

Clinical Findings

- Dense vitreous inflammation • Variable anterior chamber inflammation • Pseudohypopyon • Iris mass • Subretinal creamy yellow, elevated infiltrates of variable size • Pigmentary alterations overlying the infiltrates • Optic disc swelling from tumor infiltration of nerve or sheath • Retinal vasculitis

Ancillary Testing

- Unnecessary with known systemic lymphoma
- Fluorescein angiography is not diagnostic but often shows mottling of the RPE
- Optical coherence tomography delineates the sub-RPE location of the tumors
- Vitreous biopsy obtained from pars plana vitrectomy (the system is not primed to yield an undiluted specimen), which is then processed using flow cytometry
  - Multiple specimens may be needed to obtain a diagnosis
- Lumbar puncture
- MRI with gadolinium of the brain
- Abdominal CT
- Chest x-ray
- Bone marrow biopsy

Differential Diagnosis

- Metastatic carcinoma • Sarcoidosis • Multifocal choroiditis • Acute posterior multifocal placoid pigment epitheliopathy • Amelanotic choroidal melanoma • Acute retinal necrosis • Birdshot chorioretinopathy • Diffuse unilateral subacute neuroretinitis • Toxoplasmosis chorioretinitis • Bilateral diffuse uveal melanocytic proliferation • Leukemia • Tuberculosis • Fungal retinochoroiditis

Treatment

- Referral to a medical oncologist • Ocular irradiation • Systemic chemotherapy (intravenous and/or intrathecal)

Prognosis

- Subretinal lesions and vitreous cells respond well to treatment
  - Subretinal lesions clear with residual atrophy and vitreous cells disappear; however, recurrence within the first year is common and patients should be closely observed
- Radiation retinopathy may occur from ocular irradiation
- Overall prognosis depends on extent of systemic disease

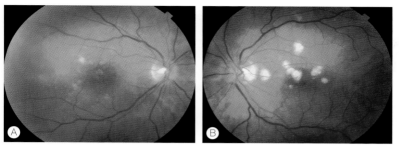

Fig. 6.15 A 58-year-old woman complaining of floaters presented with creamy, yellow subretinal spots consistent with intraocular lymphoma. Lymphoma was diagnosed with vitrectomy. Systemic work-up remains negative.

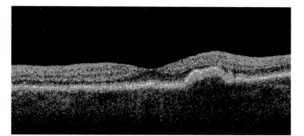

Fig. 6.16 Elevation of the lesion in the sub-RPE space is visualized on optical coherence tomography.

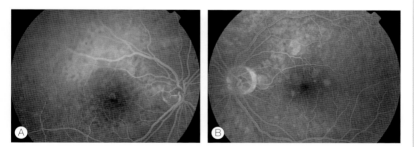

Fig. 6.17 (A) A mottled appearance on fluorescein angiography; more prominent in the right eye. (B) Staining of the subretinal infiltrates is present in the left eye.

Choroidal Osteoma

Key Facts

- Rare, benign tumor of the choroid
- Composed of bone
- Most commonly found in young women
- No racial predilection
- Sporadic inheritance
- Unilateral in 75% of cases
- Unknown pathogenesis
- No systemic manifestations

Clinical Findings

- Single lesion in juxtapapillary or peripapillary region but may occur isolated in macula
- Does not extend outside the vascular arcade
- Oval-shaped with scalloped borders
- Yellow-white to pale red color depending on amount of retinal pigment epithelium atrophy
- Minimal elevation
- May have associated shallow subretinal fluid
- Choroidal neovascularization (CNV)
- Vessels on tumor surface are short and branching
- Decalcification may occur gradually over many years

Ancillary Testing

- Fluorescein angiography shows early, patchy hyperfluorescence followed by late, intense staining of entire lesion
- Indocyanine green shows early hypofluorescence of the mass, with late generalized hyperfluorescence
- B-mode ultrasonography shows a slightly elevated, plate-like choroidal mass that is highly reflective with acoustic shadowing of the orbit
  - The acoustic shadowing may give the appearance of an optic nerve shadow
  - Persistence of the lesion occurs when the gain on the ultrasound is reduced
- A scan shows a high spike at the tumor
- CT shows a plaque in the choroid
- MRI shows a bright signal on T_1-weighted images and low intensity on T_2-weighted images

Differential Diagnosis

- Amelanotic choroidal melanoma
- Serpiginous choroidopathy
- Idiopathic sclerochoroidal calcification (multifocal, bilateral, outside vascular arcade)
- Choroidal nevus
- Choroidal metastasis
- Choroidal hemangioma
- Posterior scleritis
- Disciform scar from wet age-related macular degeneration

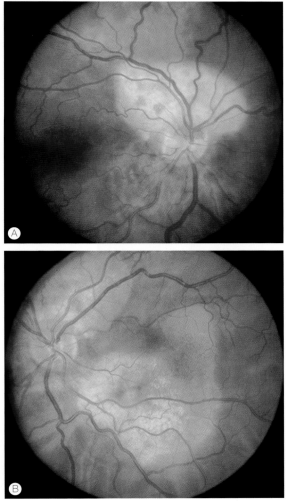

Fig. 6.18 Bilateral choroidal osteomas photographed in 1981.

Treatment

- No treatment is available for this tumor
- Treatment of CNV may include laser photocoagulation, photodynamic therapy, and anti–vascular endothelial growth factor injections

Prognosis

- Visual outcome is variable and depends on location of choroidal osteoma and presence of CNV

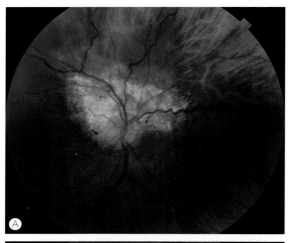

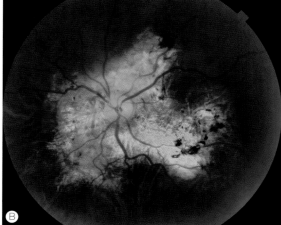

Fig. 6.19 Color photographs 24 years later of the same eyes as in Fig. 6.18. (**A,B**) Decalcification has occurred in both eyes, with residual chorioretinal atrophy. (B) The left eye has shown more growth since the initial photograph (Fig. 6.18B), with the satellite lesion along the inferior temporal arcade connecting to the optic nerve.

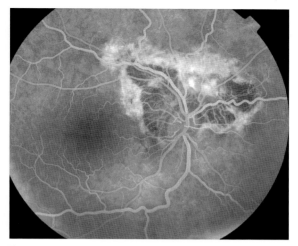

Fig. 6.20 Fluorescein angiography of the choroidal osteomas in Fig. 6.19A shows hypofluorescence in the area of choriocapillaris loss and staining of the fibrosis and edges of the lesion.

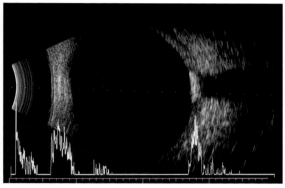

Fig. 6.21 B-mode ultrasound with increased signal of the osteoma at the level of the choroid. Acoustical shadowing mimicking an optic nerve is present.

Combined Hamartoma of the Retina and Retinal Pigment Epithelium

Key Facts

- Rare, benign, congenital retinal tumor
- Composed of retinal pigment epithelium, vessels, and glial cells
- No sexual or racial predilection
- May present at any age but most commonly in the second decade
- Associated systemically with neurofibromatosis type 2 and less commonly type 1

Clinical Findings

- Decreased visual acuity
- Slightly elevated pigmented lesions with superficial gliosis, epiretinal membrane (ERM) formation, and a fine, tortuous vascular network
- Lesions are primarily unilateral, solitary and located around optic disc, in macula, or rarely in periphery
- Retinal striae
- Exudation
- Choroidal neovascularization
- Vitreous hemorrhage
- Amblyopia
- Strabismus
- Leukocoria
- Afferent pupillary defect in extensive lesions

ancillary

Ancillary Testing

- Fluorescein angiography shows early hypofluorescence based on degree of pigmentation
  - Fluorescence occurs in arterial and venous phases, with eventual late leakage from abnormal blood vessels
- B-mode ultrasound is not beneficial—there is minimal elevation and no characteristic imaging pattern exists
- CT and MRI scans of the head are useful for imaging for the presence of bilateral acoustic neuromas

Differential Diagnosis

- Choroidal melanoma
- Choroidal nevus
- Melanocytoma
- Capillary hemangioma
- Congenital hypertrophy of the retinal pigment epithelium
- Morning glory disc anomaly
- Epiretinal membrane
- Retinoblastoma

Treatment

- Patching for amblyopia may be beneficial in selected patients
- Vitrectomy for vitreous hemorrhage
- Membrane peel may be beneficial in resolving distortion and improving vision in eyes in which the ERM is not intertwined with the retina
- Refer to primary care physician for systemic evaluation of neurofibromatosis

SECTION 6 • Tumors

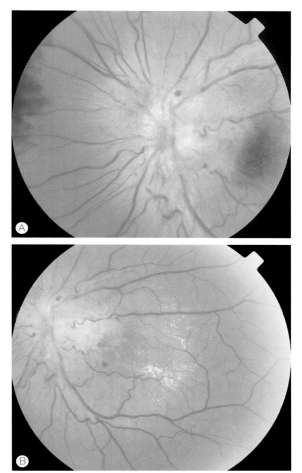

Fig. 6.22 (**A**) A combined hamartoma of the retina and retinal pigment epithelium in a 17-year-old boy who presented with a 2-year history of decreased visual acuity measuring 20/70. Gliosis, vascular tortuosity, and retinal folds are present. (**B**) Four years later, visual acuity declined to 20/400, with exudate visible in the macula.

Combined Hamartoma of the Retina and Retinal Pigment Epithelium
(Continued)

Prognosis

- Lesions usually stable and rarely progressive
- Malignant transformation has not been reported
- Visual acuity varies from 20/20 to light perception and is based on extent of optic nerve and macular involvement

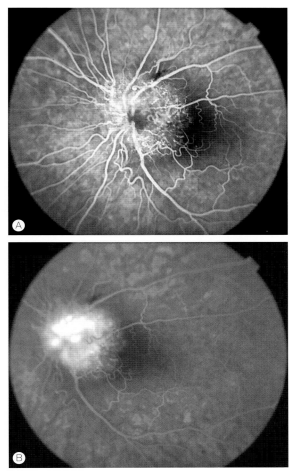

Fig. 6.23 Fluorescein angiography obtained at presentation shows (**A**) prominent vascular tortuosity with (**B**) late leakage.

Retinal Capillary Hemangioma

Key Facts

- Rare, benign vascular tumor (hamartoma) of retina or optic nerve
- No racial predilection
- Men and women equally affected
- Diagnosis made primarily in second to fourth decades
- Occurs as an isolated ocular finding (von Hippel disease) or with associated systemic manifestations in an autosomal dominant presentation (von Hippel–Lindau syndrome, VHLS)
- The exact proportion of cases that are isolated to the eye versus those cases associated with VHLS is unknown
- Patients with multiple monocular or bilateral capillary hemangiomas should be considered to have VHLS

Clinical Findings

- Red, circular tumor in peripheral retina or at optic nerve
- Tumors start as small, reddish dots and progressively enlarge
- Dilated, tortuous, and fusiform afferent artery and draining vein supply the lesion
- May be monocular or binocular and unifocal or multifocal
- Lipid exudate located around the lesion that eventually accumulates in the macula
- Subretinal fluid
- Serous retinal detachment
- Epiretinal membrane
- Retinal tears adjacent to the vascular lesion rarely occur
- Traction retinal detachment from contraction of preretinal membranes

Ancillary Testing

- Fluorescein angiography delineates the afferent arteriole, with diffuse filling and hyperfluorescence of the capillary hemangioma followed by fluorescence of the draining vein
  - Intense, late fluorescence of the lesion occurs
- Patients with suspected VHLS should undergo systemic evaluation for central nervous system hemangioblastomas, renal cell carcinoma, and pheochromocytoma

Differential Diagnosis

- Coats disease
- Arterial macroaneurysm
- Retinal cavernous hemangioma
- Retinoblastoma
- Astrocytoma

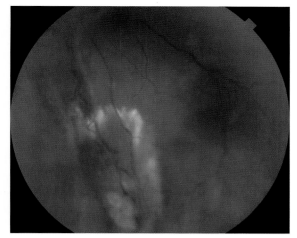

Fig. 6.24 A retinal capillary hemangioma in the peripheral retina is supplied by a tortuous artery and drained by a dilated vein. Subretinal exudate and fluid are visible in the subretinal space surrounding the vascular tumor.

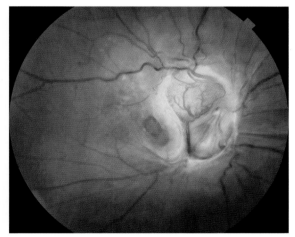

Fig. 6.25 The advanced retinal capillary hemangioma has induced traction around the optic nerve creating a macular hole. The visual acuity measures hand motions. Note the vascularity on the surface of the tumor.

Treatment

- **Laser photocoagulation is the main form of treatment:** long-duration, large spot, confluent, white burns to the lesion with scatter treatment extending beyond its borders
  - Multiple treatments are often required until the vascular tumor atrophies
- Cryopexy applied in a double freeze–thaw technique
  - Retreatment is often required at 6-week intervals until the lesion involutes and the feeder vessels return to normal
- Photodynamic therapy with verteporfin
- External beam or plaque radiation
- Pars plana vitrectomy with endolaser if multiple small vascular tumors are present
- Enucleation in blind, painful eyes

Prognosis

- Visual acuity depends on extent of macular exudation and fibrosis, with most eyes experiencing some visual loss

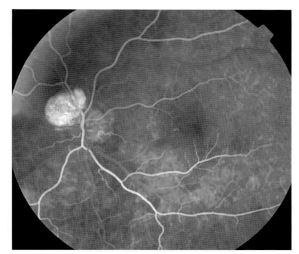

Fig. 6.26 Fluorescence of an isolated retinal capillary hemangioma of the optic nerve. No other vascular tumors were identified in either eye.

Retinal Cavernous Hemangioma

Key Facts

- Benign vascular tumor of the retina
- Similar vascular changes may concomitantly occur cutaneously or in the central nervous system (CNS)
- Classified as a phakomatoses
- Patients may be asymptomatic or present with a decline in visual acuity
- Inheritance is usually sporadic
  - a small minority of patients may have a dominantly inherited form as part of an oculoneurocutaneous syndrome

Clinical Findings

- Cluster of dark, grape-like, variable-sized aneurysms arising from a retinal venule
- Lesions may occur anywhere within the retina or adjacent to optic disc
- Vast majority of lesions are stable but minority may show slow progression
- White fibrous tissue within vascular cluster
- Retinal traction (rare)
- Vitreous hemorrhage (rare)

Ancillary Testing

- Testing is rarely required—diagnosis is typically made through clinical examination
- Fluorescein angiography is the most useful diagnostic test
  - Arterial phase: vascular channels are hypofluorescent
  - Venous and recirculation phases: fluorescein accumulates and fluoresces within the vascular aneurysms without evidence of leakage; the dependent blood within the vascular spaces creates a distinctive blood–fluorescein interface
- B-scan ultrasonography may be useful when a vitreous hemorrhage is present
  - The scan shows a defined surface without choroidal shadowing or excavation
- A scan of the lesion shows a high initial spike followed by high internal reflectivity
- Systemic evaluation by a primary care physician if cutaneous or CNS lesions are suspected

Differential Diagnosis

- Retinal capillary hemangioma
- Coats disease
- Branch retinal vein occlusion

Treatment

- Observation—lesions are typically non-progressive
- If vitreous hemorrhage occurs, lesions may be treated with laser photocoagulation, cryotherapy, or plaque radiotherapy
  - The overall value of these treatments is unknown
- Pars plana vitrectomy in conjunction with laser or cryotherapy should be considered in more extensive non-clearing vitreous hemorrhage

Prognosis

- Typically good visual outcome unless the lesion is in the macula or macular traction occurs

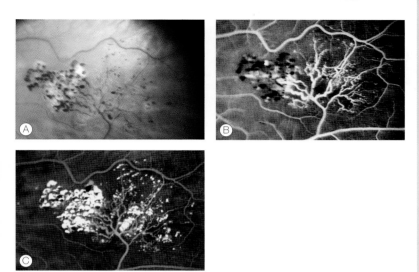

Fig. 6.27 (**A**) Color photograph of a retinal cavernous hemangioma in the peripheral retina. Accompanying fluorescein angiography shows (**B**) progressive accumulation of fluorescein within the vascular spaces, with (**C**) an eventual blood-fluorescein interface present.

Retinal Astrocytic Hamartoma

Key Facts

- Benign tumor arising from glial cells within the retina
- Occurs as an isolated, acquired, sporadic ocular finding (retinal astrocytoma) or more commonly as a congenital tumor associated with tuberous sclerosis (astrocytic hamartoma)
- Tumor progression is uncommon in congenital astrocytic hamartoma
  - acquired astrocytomas are more aggressive and may show progressive growth
- Tuberous sclerosis is autosomal dominant, with an incidence of 1 in 15 000 to 1 in 100 000
- Nearly 50% of all patients with tuberous sclerosis develop astrocytic hamartomas
- Hemorrhage and subretinal fluid are more common in acquired astrocytomas

Clinical Findings

- **Lesions clinically present in two forms:**
  - Yellow-white, ovoid or circular mulberry-like elevations of the retina with varying degrees of calcification • Small, flat, smooth lesions without calcification
- Vitreous hemorrhage (rare)
- Subretinal hemorrhage (rare)
- Retinal detachment (rare)
- **Systemic findings of tuberous sclerosis include:**
  - hypopigmented ashen leaf spots on trunk and limbs • adenoma sebaceum in a butterfly pattern over cheeks, chin, and forehead • yellowish thickening of skin over lumbosacral region (shagreen patch) • subungual fibromas • seizures (90% incidence) • mental retardation (60% incidence) • cardiac rhabdomyoma • angioleiomyomas of kidney, liver, pancreas, and adrenal glands • calcified nodules along ventricles of brain

Ancillary Testing

- Tumor is hypofluorescent on fluorescein angiography in arterial phase
  - fine vessels surrounding the tumor leak profusely, causing hyperfluorescence during venous phase
- A-scan shows high internal reflectivity
- B-scan ultrasound shows a well-demarcated lesion with occasional acoustic shadowing
- Fine needle aspiration may be needed in cases in which the diagnosis is in doubt
- CT scan of the brain for evidence of calcified nodules along the ventricles
- A primary care physician should evaluate patients and their family members for evidence of tuberous sclerosis

Differential Diagnosis

- Retinoblastoma • Amelanotic choroidal melanoma • Myelinated nerve fiber layer • Retinal capillary hemangioma • Choroidal or retinal granuloma • Optic disc drusen

Treatment

- Observation, because most lesions are stable and show no growth • Grid laser photocoagulation to areas of exudative retinal detachment while avoiding the tumor to stimulate reabsorbtion of fluid

Prognosis

- Good visual prognosis
- When severe epilepsy and seizures are present, death usually occurs by third decade

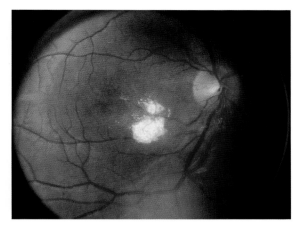

Fig. 6.28 A girl with tuberous sclerosis and 20/100 visual acuity presented with a whitish yellow mulberry-shaped tumor in the macula consistent with an astrocytic hamartoma. Of her two sisters, one had a similar retinal tumor, while one had a normal retinal examination.

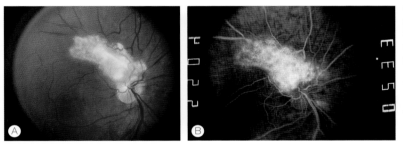

Fig. 6.29 (A) Color photograph of an astrocytic hamartoma along the superior temporal arcade adjacent to the optic nerve. The tumor shows (B) fine surface vessels in the arteriovenous phase that begin to leak, with extensive leakage visible in the venous phase of the angiogram.

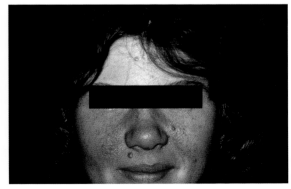

Fig. 6.30 Facial photograph of the patient from Fig. 6.29, showing adenoma sebaceum.

Section 7
Retinal Detachment and Allied Diseases

Lattice Degeneration

Key Facts

- Found in 6–10% of the general population
- No sexual predilection
- Bilateral in ≤50% of patients
- Variable clinical presentations
- Found in 30% of all eyes with rhegmatogenous retinal detachments

Clinical Findings

- Linear pigmentation anterior to the equator that may span multiple clock hours
- Lattice lesions may run parallel to one another in same quadrant
- Sclerotic vessels
- Branching white lines
- Chorioretinal atrophy
- Retinal hole
- Retinal tear
- Acute or chronic retinal detachment

Ancillary Testing

- None

Differential Diagnosis

- Cobblestone degeneration
- Retinoschisis
- Chorioretinal scar
- Peripheral cystoid degeneration

Treatment

- Prophylactic laser of asymptomatic lattice degeneration with or without atrophic retinal holes is not recommended, because the risk of retinal detachment is low
- Laser retinopexy for retinal tears
- Laser demarcation for subclinical acute or chronic retinal detachment
- Pneumatic retinopexy, scleral buckle, or vitrectomy with or without scleral buckle for rhegmatogenous retinal detachment

Prognosis

- 1% risk of retinal detachment in all eyes with lattice degeneration over a 10-year period

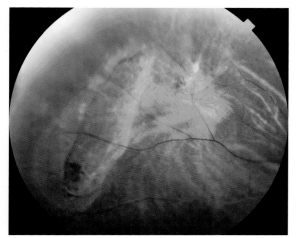

Fig. 7.1 Lattice degeneration with branching white lines.

Retinal Tear

Key Facts

- Full-thickness break in neurosensory retina
- Vitreous traction is most common cause
- Incidence increases with age
- Men and women equally affected
- Risk factors include myopia, lattice degeneration, and trauma
- Patients present with new onset floaters (from vitreous hemorrhage or vitreous detachment) and photopsias (from vitreoretinal traction)
- Retinal tears can be associated systemically with Marfan, Stickler, Wagner, and Ehlers–Danlos syndromes as well as homocystinuria
- Goal of treatment is to create a chorioretinal adhesion around the tear to prevent vitreous fluid from entering the subretinal space and creating a retinal detachment

Clinical Findings

- Horseshoe-shaped tear with or without surrounding subretinal fluid
- Tear usually occurs at the vitreous base but may occur near equator
- Giant retinal tears extend three or more clock hours
- Vitreous hemorrhage
- Posterior vitreous detachment
- Pigmentation surrounding tears when chronic
- Vitreous traction
- Lattice degeneration

Ancillary Testing

- Clinical examination alone usually sufficient
- Ultrasound to evaluate for retinal tear and/or detachment when vitreous hemorrhage prevents visualization of retina

Differential Diagnosis

- Operculated hole
- Atrophic hole
- Paving stone degeneration
- Chorioretinal scar
- Peripheral cystoid degeneration
- Venous occlusive disease with neovascularization causing vitreous hemorrhage

Treatment

- Laser photocoagulation to surround retinal tear with a minimum of three concentric rows of laser
- Cryopexy around retinal tear
- **Observation if:**
  - tear is chronic • tear demarcated by pigmentation • absence of vitreous traction or surrounding subretinal fluid • patient is asymptomatic

Prognosis

- Tears treated with laser photocoagulation or cryopexy rarely progress to retinal detachments
- Symptomatic retinal tears, if untreated, will lead to retinal detachment in about one-third of eyes
- Epiretinal membrane can form in ≤5% of eyes with retinal tears

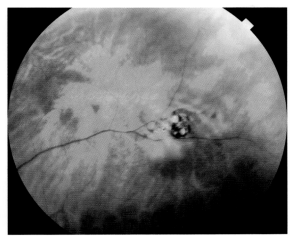

Fig. 7.2 A posterior retinal tear with an avulsed retinal flap. Shallow subretinal fluid is present at the temporal edge of the tear. Laser photocoagulation was performed.

Degenerative Adult Retinoschisis

Key Facts

- Peripheral retinal degeneration
- Patients typically asymptomatic
- Splitting of the retina at outer plexiform or inner nuclear layer
- Neurons are severed, with loss of visual function in the involved retina
- Inferior temporal quadrant is most commonly affected site
- Usually bilateral and symmetric
- No sexual or racial predilection
- Retinal breaks occur in outer retinal layer in about 15% of patients but rarely occur in inner retina

Clinical Findings

- Smooth, convex elevation of peripheral retina
- Whitish flecks may be present on inner retinal surface
- Sheathing of vessels in the schisis cavity may be present
- Inner retina may be thin and nearly transparent
- Retinal breaks in outer or inner retinal layer
- Absence of a demarcation line
- Retinal detachment is rare and may be localized with outer retinal breaks or progressive with outer and inner retinal breaks

Ancillary Testing

- Visual field testing shows an absolute scotoma
- Splitting of the neurosensory retina is present on optical coherence tomography

Differential Diagnosis

- Rhegmatogenous retinal detachment
- Non-rhegmatogenous retinal detachment
- Central serous retinopathy
- Choroidal melanoma

Treatment

- Observation in vast majority of cases
- Laser demarcation of the schisis cavity is of no benefit
- Surgical repair of rhegmatogenous retinal detachment by pneumatic retinopexy, pars plana vitrectomy, or scleral buckle

Prognosis

- Retinoschisis cavities may show slow enlargement but usually do not progress
- Involvement of the macula is rare
- Visual outcome is excellent, with the vast majority of patients unaware of the presence of retinoschisis
- Most retinal detachments are localized schisis-related detachments that do not progress

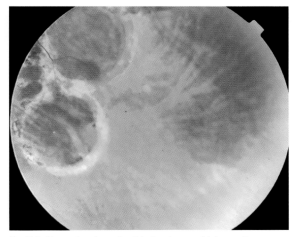

Fig. 7.3 Round outer retinal holes in a schisis cavity.

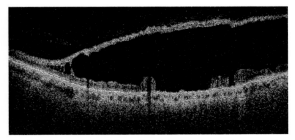

Fig. 7.4 Separation of the retina into two layers is present on optical coherence tomography.

Rhegmatogenous Retinal Detachment

Key Facts

- Caused by vitreous traction exerted on a full-thickness retinal defect, allowing liquefied vitreous fluid to enter the subretinal space
- Photopsias and floaters are early symptoms
- Patients may be asymptomatic until the macula is involved
- **Risk factors include:**
  - myopia • retinal detachment in opposite eye • trauma • lattice degeneration • acute posterior vitreous detachment (PVD) • pseudophakia • aphakia • Nd : YAG laser capsulotomy
- 1 in 10 000 risk

Clinical Findings

- Decreased visual acuity • PVD with liquefaction of vitreous • Pigment or hemorrhage in vitreous cavity • Elevation of the retina, with fluid separating the neurosensory retina from the retinal pigment epithelium • Corrugated appearance to the retina in more acute detachments, smooth elevation with thinning in more chronic detachments • Retinal tears primarily occurring in the vitreous base

Ancillary Testing

- Ultrasound when vitreous hemorrhage prevents direct visualization of retina

Differential Diagnosis

- Retinoschisis • Exudative retinal detachment • Traction retinal detachment • Choroidal neoplasm

Treatment

- The goal of treatment is to seal the retinal break to prevent further fluid accumulation under the retina
  - Relief of the vitreous traction is usually necessary
- Surgical intervention should be performed promptly to maximize visual recovery
- Chronic, subclinical retinal detachments with a demarcation line in the inferior retina not involving the macula may be observed
- Argon laser photocoagulation may be used to demarcate limited subclinical retinal detachments in superior retina and asymptomatic chronic detachments without demarcation lines in inferior retina
- Pneumatic retinopexy for retinal detachments with one or more breaks within one or two clock hours of one another occurring in the superior eight clock hours of the eye
  - Positioning for 3–4 days is then required to position the intraocular gas over the retinal tear for tamponade • Rarely, inferior detachments can be treated with pneumatic retinopexy and head-down positioning
- Scleral buckle (segmental or encircling) with cryopexy to retinal tears and gas tamponade with or without external drainage of subretinal fluid
- Pars plana vitrectomy with endolaser surrounding retinal tears and intravitreal gas tamponade, either alone or with an encircling scleral band

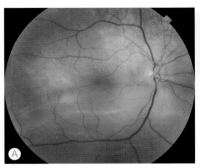
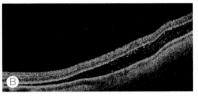

Fig. 7.5 (**A**) Inferior rhegmatogenous retinal detachment with subretinal fluid splitting the fovea. (**B**) Optical coherence tomography shows separation of the retinal pigment epithelium from the neurosensory retina.

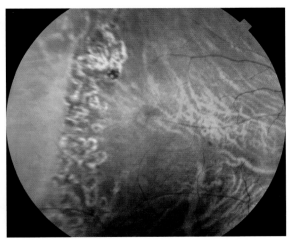

Fig. 7.6 Laser demarcation of a chronic temporal retinal detachment.

Prognosis

- Visual outcome, regardless of method of treatment, depends primarily on preoperative visual acuity
- **Other factors limiting postoperative visual recovery include:**
  - formation of proliferative vitreoretinopathy • epiretinal membrane • cystoid macular edema • macular atrophy
- Untreated retinal detachments involving the fovea will lead to diminished vision in all cases
- Laser demarcation of subclinical retinal detachments has a high success rate, with few cases requiring more definitive surgical treatment
- Pneumatic retinopexy is successful in 80% or more of all eyes
- Scleral buckle surgery has a nearly 85–90% anatomical success rate with one operation
- Pars plana vitrectomy is successful in >90% of eyes with one operation
- Overall, the anatomical success rate for repairing rhegmatogenous retinal detachments is 98%

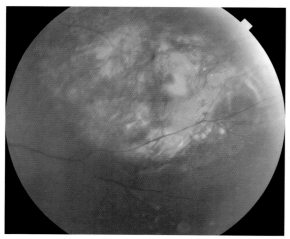

Fig. 7.7 Chorioretinal scar formation surrounding a retinal tear in an eye 7 days after pneumatic retinopexy.

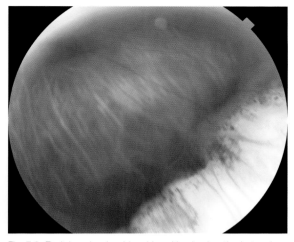

Fig. 7.8 Peripheral scleral buckle with chorioretinal atrophy 1 year after retinal detachment repair.

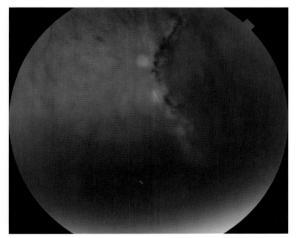

Fig. 7.9 A pigmented demarcation line in the inferior temporal quadrant of a patient with a subclinical retinal detachment. The detachment has been present for 9 years without any evidence of progression, and the patient remains asymptomatic.

Proliferative Vitreoretinopathy

Key Facts

- Retinal pigment epithelium cells released during a retinal tear migrate on to retinal and vitreous surfaces, creating a cellular membrane that subsequently contracts leading to a traction retinal detachment
- One of the leading causes of failure of retinal detachment surgery
  - new or missed retinal breaks are the leading cause of recurrent detachments
- Affects ≤5–10% of all retinal detachments
- No sexual predilection

Clinical Findings

- Retinal detachment with stiff-appearing retina that does not undulate
- Funnel retinal detachment
- Retinal tears with rolled edges
- Epiretinal membrane
- Pigment on retinal surface
- Star folds from membrane contraction
- Subretinal bands
- Pigment dispersed in vitreous cavity
- Neovascularization of iris
- Hypotony from traction on ciliary body

Ancillary Testing

- Ultrasound required only if there is no view to the retina
  - Ultrasound shows a retinal detachment with limited mobility or retina in a funnel configuration

Differential Diagnosis

- Exudative retinal detachment
- Traction retinal detachment from diabetes or retinopathy of prematurity

Treatment

- **Surgical management includes:**
  - pars plana vitrectomy with or without scleral buckle • removal of subretinal and epiretinal membranes • retinectomy to relieve retinal traction when required • endolaser • perfluorocarbon liquid and tamponade with long-acting gas (C_3F_8) or silicone oil

Prognosis

- Surgical success for retinal reattachment approaches 80%
- Often more than one surgical procedure is required to reattach the retina
- Visual recovery limited and typically poor, with acuity measuring 20/400 or less

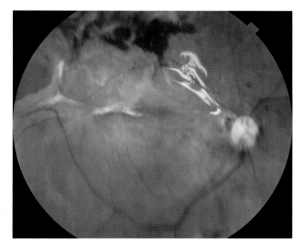

Fig. 7.10 A persistent traction retinal detachment in an eye filled with silicone oil (shimmering light reflex in the macula). The macula is out of focus, as the subretinal band in the temporal macula extending to the fovea is elevating the retina. Heavy laser scar is present superiorly to the macula.

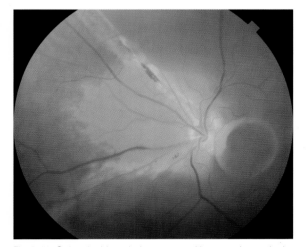

Fig. 7.11 Subretinal bands in an eye with a traction retinal detachment. A circular subretinal band is present temporal to the disc.

Non-rhegmatogenous (Exudative) Retinal Detachment

Key Facts

- Elevation of retina from accumulation of fluid, exudate, or blood in the subretinal space in the absence of retinal break or traction
- **The pathophysiology includes:**
  - breakdown of the blood–retinal barrier (e.g. central serous retinopathy, Harada disease)
  - an increase in fluid flow into the subretinal space (e.g. choroidal tumors, malignant hypertension) and/or impairment in outflow of fluid from the eye (e.g. scleritis) combined with inability of the retinal pigment epithelium to pump fluid out of the subretinal space

Clinical Findings

- Smooth and convex elevation of the retina
- Detachment may be limited and localized to the macula or may be bullous and extend to the ora serrata
- When bullous, fluid tends to shift on changes in head positioning
- Absence of a retinal tear
- Fluid in subretinal space may be proteinaceous, serous (clear or turbid), or hemorrhagic
- Ocular signs such as redness or pain vary depending on underlying etiology

Ancillary Testing

- Fluorescein angiography to show focal areas of choroidal or retinal leakage
- **Ultrasound to image:**
  - the subretinal space for presence of tumors • a thickened choroid in inflammatory disorders • the retina when vitreous hemorrhage present
- Optical coherence tomography to evaluate and follow shallow neurosensory detachments
- CT or MRI when orbital pathology suspected
- Hematologic evaluation of systemic inflammatory disorders

Differential Diagnosis

- Rhegmatogenous retinal detachment
- Retinoschisis
- Choroidal effusion
- Suprachoroidal hemorrhage
- Choroidal tumor

Treatment

- Treat any underlying systemic or ocular condition

Prognosis

- Visual outcome depends on underlying cause of exudative retinal detachment

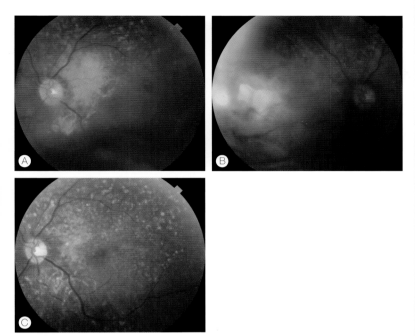

Fig. 7.12 (**A**) A bullous exudative retinal detachment involving the fovea is present inferiorly and temporally in an eye with exudative AMD. (**B**) A nasal view of the retina shows the subretinal hemorrhage and exudates from the peripheral choroidal neovascularization causing the non-rhegmatogenous detachment. (**C**) An attached retina and diffuse drusen from the same eye 6 months before the photographs taken in (A) and (B).

Choroidal Hemorrhage

Key Facts

- Hemorrhage in suprachoroidal space • Severe complication of most ocular surgeries • Varies from a limited, asymptomatic hemorrhage to a massive bleed with possible expulsion of intraocular contents • Hemorrhaging occurs at time of surgery or may be delayed by 1–2 weeks • Etiology is typically from a rapid decline in IOP (e.g. following a surgical incision), causing a vessel in the eye wall to rupture
- **Common procedures causing choroidal hemorrhage are:**
  - penetrating keratoplasty (0.4%) • glaucoma filtering procedures (0.73%) • cataract surgery (0.2%)
- **Systemic risk factors include:**
  - advancing age • hypertension • arteriosclerosis • anticoagulant use
- **Ocular risk factors include:**
  - high myopia • glaucoma • vitreous removal or loss • retinal laser photocoagulation • previous eye surgery
- Males and females equally affected

Clinical Findings

- Smooth brown elevation of the choroid and retina • Hemorrhage anterior to the equator may expand circumferentially • Postequatorial hemorrhages tend to be unilobular or multilobular • Kissing choroidals occur when opposing eye walls touch in the central vitreous cavity from extensive hemorrhage • Loss of red reflex • Breakthrough vitreous hemorrhage • Flat anterior chamber • Elevated IOP • Severe ocular pain • Iris, vitreous, or retinal incarceration in surgical wounds • Rhegmatogenous retinal detachment

Ancillary tests

- B-mode ultrasound of choroidal detachment shows smooth, dome-shaped elevation that does not undulate
  - A recent hemorrhage has a solid appearance that is highly reflective • Over time, the blood liquefies and the suprachoroidal space has low reflectivity
- On A scan, the hemorrhage has a medium to high internal reflectivity
- Choroidal hemorrhages fail to transilluminate light

Differential Diagnosis

- Choroidal effusion • Choroidal melanoma • Metastatic tumor • Retinal detachment

Treatment

- Observation for limited choroidal hemorrhages • Drainage of suprachoroidal hemorrhage via posterior sclerotomy is considered when there are kissing choroidals or persistent shallowing of the anterior chamber
  - If clinical circumstances allow, surgery should be delayed 10–14 days to allow for liquefaction of the blood to ensure a more complete drainage
- Pars plana vitrectomy for non-clearing vitreous hemorrhage • Pars plana vitrectomy with long-acting gas or silicone oil tamponade when rhegmatogenous retinal detachment present • Immediate closure of surgical wound if choroidal hemorrhage suspected or visualized or if there is a change in the red reflex

Prognosis

- Limited suprachoroidal hemorrhages have a good prognosis because the blood reabsorbs over 1–2 months without affecting visual acuity • More severe hemorrhages have a variable visual outcome
  - Presence of kissing choroidals does not necessarily portend a poor visual outcome
- The effectiveness of posterior sclerotomy on visual outcome is unknown • Presence of an incarceration of intraocular contents or a rhegmatogenous retinal detachment carries a poor visual outcome

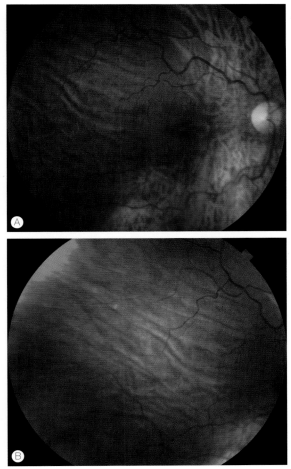

Fig. 7.13 An asymptomatic patient 4 weeks removed from uncomplicated phacoemulsification surgery was referred for evaluation of a choroidal melanoma. (**A**) A limited suprachoroidal hemorrhage is visible just temporal to the fovea as an isolated, shallow, brown elevation of the retina and choroid. (**B**) A more temporal photograph of the lesion.

Congenital Optic Disc Pit

Key Facts

- Unknown pathogenesis
- Occurs in about 1 in 11 000 patients
- No associated systemic abnormalities
- 95% of pits are unilateral
- Subretinal fluid originates from vitreous cavity or subarachnoid space

Clinical Findings

- Oval or round depression of the optic disc that is gray or yellow in appearance
- 50% of pits are located at the temporal edge of the disc, with one-third located centrally
- Multiple pits may be identified on the same disc
- Shallow retinal detachment confined to the macula in 40% of eyes
- Macular hole
- Enlargement of the affected optic disc compared with the normal contralateral disc
- Peripapillary pigmentary changes
- Peripapillary choroidal neovascularization (rare)

Ancillary Testing

- Optical coherence tomography to evaluate the presence of a retinal detachment and schisis cavity
- **Visual field defects include:**
  - enlarged blind spot • central scotoma from macular retinal detachment
    - field defects from the pit that may mimic glaucomatous field defects

Differential Diagnosis

- Central serous retinopathy
- Optic nerve coloboma
- Morning glory disc

Treatment

- Observation
- When visual acuity is declining, laser photocoagulation is an initial treatment of choice
  - Laser burns are placed in two or three rows at the edge of the optic disc, adjacent to the optic pit and in the area of retina detachment, extending superiorly and inferiorly into normal retina • The goal of laser is to create a barrier that blocks fluid from entering the subretinal space through the pit
    - If this fails, a second application may be applied a few months after the initial treatment
- Pars plana vitrectomy with elevation of the posterior hyaloid, peripapillary laser, and gas tamponade

Prognosis

- Nearly 40% of optic pits are associated with retinal detachments
- Rarely, the retinal detachment will resolve spontaneously
- Persistent retinal detachment results in 20/200 or worse visual acuity
- Presence of a macular hole has a poor visual prognosis
- No formal clinical trials have evaluated the effects of treatment
- Laser may be effective in ≥50% of eyes
- Resolution of the neurosensory detachment following treatment may take 3–6 months or more given the chronic nature of the subretinal fluid

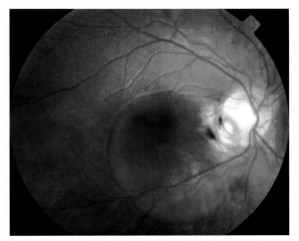

Fig. 7.14 A gray optic disc pit with peripapillary scar from previous laser. A retinal detachment confined to the macula is present.

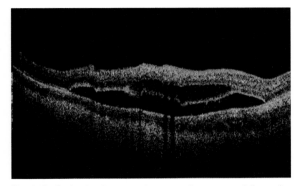

Fig. 7.15 Optical coherence tomography scanned through the macula of the patient in Fig. 7.14, showing a combination of a schisis cavity and a neurosensory detachment.

Section 8

Vitreous

Asteroid Hyalosis

Key Facts

- Benign condition
- Unknown etiology
- Occurs in middle age or later
- Identified in <0.05% of general population
- Affects males greater than females by a 2 : 1 margin
- Unilateral in 75% of cases
- Possible rare association with diabetes

Clinical Findings

- Yellow-white opacities in the vitreous body of varying densities
- Visualization of retina may be difficult
- In eyes with posterior vitreous detachment, asteroid bodies remain only within vitreous gel

Ancillary Testing

- Fluorescein angiography allows better visualization of the retina—the fluorescence from the activated dye originates from the retina and is projected into the camera, creating an image unimpeded by vitreous opacities
  - Color photography is difficult—the flash from the camera reflects off the asteroid bodies

Differential Diagnosis

- Cholesterolosis
- Amyloidosis
- Chronic vitreous hemorrhage
- Chronic vitritis

Treatment

- **Pars plana vitrectomy only in rare cases when:**
  - asteroid hyalosis causes visual symptoms
  - clinical examination and treatment of retina are obstructed by dense asteroid hyalosis (i.e. proliferative diabetic retinopathy)

Prognosis

- Rarely leads to visual disturbance

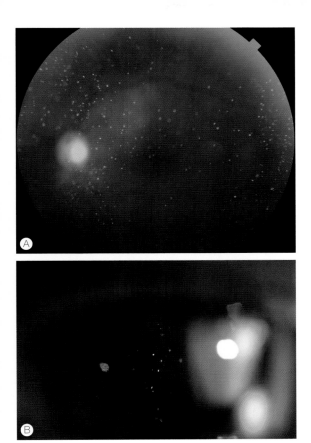

Fig. 8.1 (**A**) Small yellow-white bodies imaged in the
midvitreous of an eye with asteroid hyalosis. (**B**) A
slit-lamp view shows the asteroid bodies in the anterior
vitreous behind the lens.

Section 9

Macular Diseases

Epiretinal Membrane

Key Facts

- Transparent fibrocellular proliferation on inner retinal surface
- **Occurs from:**
  - posterior vitreous detachment • after retinal detachment repair • uveitis
    - retinal tears • branch vein occlusion
- Retinal traction leads to retinal thickening, causing varying levels of decreased vision with or without metamorphopsia
- Visual decline will often reach a plateau without any further change
- Patients may have significant visual symptoms of metamorphopsia despite good visual acuity

Clinical Findings

- Variable depending on degree and thickness of membrane • Retinal striae and folds • Dragging and tortuosity of retinal vessels • Distortion of retinal anatomy in macula • Macular edema • Macular hole • Partial-thickness macular hole

Ancillary Testing

- Optical coherence tomography is the best test to evaluate epiretinal membranes
  - The membrane is a highly reflective yellow-red layer on the inner retina, with retinal thickening • Cystic spaces in the retina identified as black hyporeflective circles may be present • Any vitreoretinal traction is identified, and pseudoholes appear as partial-thickness holes with an intact photoreceptor layer
- Fluorescein angiography (FA) will identify areas of leakage, if present, but is not necessary in making the clinical diagnosis
- Amsler grid testing shows metamorphopsia

Differential Diagnosis

- Vitreomacular traction syndrome • Postoperative cystoid macular edema
  - Macular hole

Treatment

- For patients with minimal visual loss and no metamorphopsia, observation is advised because visual decline tends to plateau and stabilize • Pars plana vitrectomy with membrane peel is offered when significant visual loss and disabling metamorphopsia are present

Prognosis

- Degree of visual decline and metamorphopsia depends on thickness of membrane and degree of retinal distortion and macular edema
  - Thicker membranes induce more retinal distortion and lead to greater visual decline • Thinner, cellophane-like membranes with minimal retinal changes may not affect visual acuity
- Visual acuity usually remains stable following diagnosis
- After pars plana vitrectomy, 60–85% of eyes gain two or more Snellen lines, with improvement of metamorphopsia in most cases
  - Visual improvement often takes 2–3 months after surgery to improve
    - Macular edema and retinal thickening also improve in most cases after membrane peel • Visual acuity rarely returns to normal

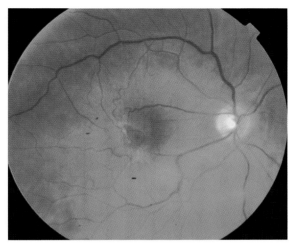

Fig. 9.1 An epiretinal membrane with distortion of the macula. Retinal vessels are pulled centrally toward the preretinal fibrosis localized over the fovea.

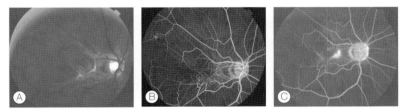

Fig. 9.2 (**A**) A prominent epiretinal membrane on red-free photograph. (**B**) On FA, the vasculature is distorted by the epiretinal membrane, with (**C**) leakage in the late phase of the angiogram.

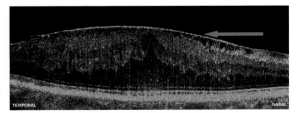

Fig. 9.3 The epiretinal membrane on this optical coherence tomography image is the reflective band on the inner retina (arrow).

Chorioretinal Folds

Key Facts

- Caused by a reduction in the surface area of the inner sclera, throwing the inner choroid and outer retina into fine folds
- Clinical symptoms from the folds rarely occur
- Most cases are idiopathic, occurring in males with 1–6 D of hyperopia
- Idiopathic folds are usually bilateral and symmetric
- **Other etiologies causing monocular folds include:**
  - orbital tumors
  - scleral buckle
  - scleritis
  - orbital inflammatory syndrome
  - thyroid eye disease
  - choroidal neovascularization
  - hypotony
  - optic disc swelling

Clinical Findings

- Alternating light and dark lines in the retina, usually running parallel to one another
- Folds are typically in a horizontal, vertical, or oblique fashion but may also radiate outward from a central point
- Macula is the most common location

Ancillary Testing

- Fluorescein angiography shows alternating light and dark lines
  - The crest of the fold has attenuated retinal pigment epithelium (RPE) and transmits fluorescence, while the trough of the fold has thicker RPE and blocks fluorescence
- Ultrasound may identify flattening of the posterior sclera
- Imaging of the orbit with MRI or CT if an orbital tumor is suspected
- Thyroid function tests if thyroid eye disease is suspected

Differential Diagnosis

- Epiretinal membrane
- Retinal detachment with proliferative vitreoretinopathy and retinal folds

Treatment

- No treatment exists for idiopathic chorioretinal folds
- Any identifiable underlying cause of the chorioretinal folds (i.e. orbital tumor) should be treated

Prognosis

- Most patients with idiopathic chorioretinal folds are asymptomatic and require routine examinations
- In eyes with a known cause of the chorioretinal folds, removal of the inciting agent will lead to resolution

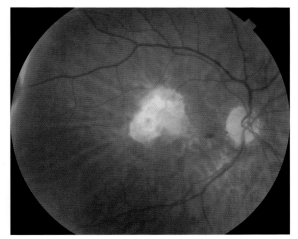

Fig. 9.4 Chorioretinal folds radiate outward due to contraction from a fibrotic choroidal neovascular membrane.

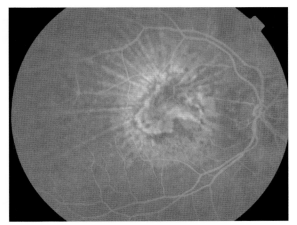

Fig. 9.5 Fluorescein angiogram of the color photograph in Fig. 9.4, showing alternating dark and light bands from the chorioretinal folds. Staining of the fibrotic choroidal neovascularization is present.

Partial-thickness Macular Hole

Key Facts

- Macular hole with tissue loss in inner retina while photoreceptor layer remains intact
- No racial or sexual predominance
- Minimal visual disturbance

Clinical Findings

- Oval-shaped defect at the fovea
- Epiretinal membrane (ERM)
- Posterior vitreous detachment

Ancillary Testing

- Optical coherence tomography reveals a retinal defect of the inner retina while sparing the photoreceptor layer

Differential Diagnosis

- Full-thickness macular hole
- ERM
- Vitreomacular traction syndrome

Treatment

- Observation
- Pars plana vitrectomy with membrane peel may be considered if an ERM is present and causing distortion

Prognosis

- Vision may be slightly declined but typically remains stable in the 20/25 to 20/50 range

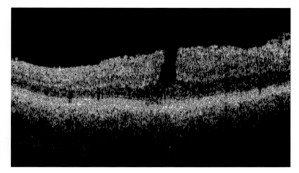

Fig. 9.6 A partial-thickness macular hole as viewed by optical coherence tomography. Compared with a full-thickness macular hole, the photoreceptors are preserved in a partial-thickness hole.

Macular Hole

Key Facts

- Full-thickness defect of neurosensory retina in the macula involving the fovea
- Central scotoma with metamorphopsia and decreased vision
- Females affected more commonly than males
- Mean age of onset around 60 years
- Typically monocular
- Etiology is abnormal vitreous traction on the fovea
- **Rarely due to:**
  - trauma • diabetic retinopathy • post retinal detachment • hypertensive retinopathy • optic pit • lightning strike

Clinical Findings

- **Stage 1 macular hole:** detachment of the photoreceptors without a full-thickness defect
  - A posterior vitreous detachment (PVD) is not present • Subdivided into stage 1a and 1b macular holes • A yellow spot is clinically visible in stage 1a macular holes • A yellow ring in the fovea is present in a stage 1b macular hole
- **Stage 2:** full-thickness macular hole <400 μm in diameter without a PVD
  - The full-thickness retinal defect is either central or eccentric, with the vitreous remaining inserted on to the macular hole flap
- **Stage 3:** full-thickness macular hole >400 μm in diameter without a PVD
- **Stage 4:** full-thickness macular hole >400 μm in diameter, clinically similar to a stage 3 hole but a PVD is present
- In stages 2–4, a circumferential cuff of subretinal fluid surrounds the macular hole, except in some chronic stage 4 holes
- Punctate yellow spots are present at the level of the retinal pigment epithelium in more chronic holes
- Epiretinal membrane (ERM) may or may not be present

Ancillary Testing

- Optical coherence tomography (OCT) accurately views the vitreoretinal interface and creates a cross-sectional image of the retina that accurately diagnoses a stage 1–4 macular hole
  - Take care to ensure that the OCT scan is centered on the fovea—off-centered scans may miss the hole, creating instead a scan of a neurosensory detachment with cystoid macular edema
- Fluorescein angiography is not generally beneficial in diagnosing a macular hole but is useful in excluding other diagnoses

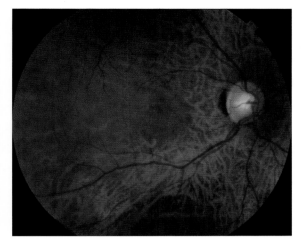

Fig. 9.7 Full-thickness macular hole.

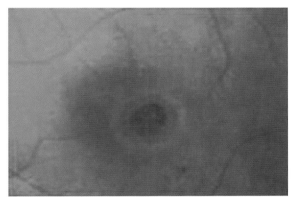

Fig. 9.8 Magnified view of a macular hole with a cuff of surrounding subretinal fluid.

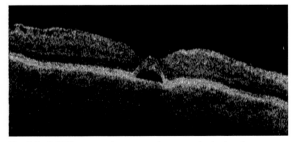

Fig. 9.9 OCT image of a stage 1a macular hole. A neurosensory detachment is visible with a foveal contour still intact. There is no full-thickness defect.

Differential Diagnosis

- ERM with macular pseudohole
- Lamellar hole
- Cystoid macular edema
- Vitreomacular traction syndrome
- Central serous retinopathy

Treatment

- **Stage 1:** generally observed because nearly 50% spontaneously resolve
- **Stages 2–4:** pars plana vitrectomy, peeling of the posterior hyaloid, and intravitreal injection of a long-acting gas (SF_6 or C_3F_8), followed by face-down positioning for 5–7 days

Prognosis

- Without treatment, vision generally stabilizes around 20/400
- About 10–15% of patients develop a macular hole in the other eye
- Vitrectomy is successful in closing 90% of all macular holes, with about two-thirds of eyes improving two or more Snellen acuity lines
- Factors that improve surgical outcome include smaller size of the macular hole and better preoperative visual acuity

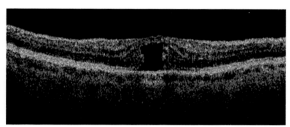

Fig. 9.10 A stage 1b macular hole on OCT. The photoreceptor layer is elevated and split centrally, while the inner retina is still intact.

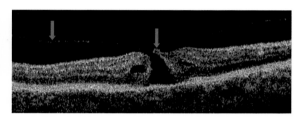

Fig. 9.11 A full-thickness stage 2 macular hole with an eccentric hole and persistent attachment of the vitreous to the retina (red arrows).

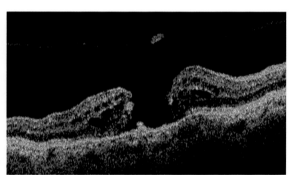

Fig. 9.12 A stage 4 macular hole is imaged on OCT with complete separation of the posterior vitreous hyaloid and an overlying operculum. Not that there is only bare retinal pigment epithelium present at the base of the OCT.

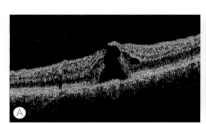
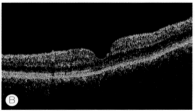

Fig. 9.13 (**A**) Preoperative OCT of a woman with a stage 2 macular hole. (**B**) Three weeks after vitrectomy, membrane peel, and 25% SF$_6$ gas tamponade with face-down positioning, there is closure of the macular hole and restoration of a normal foveal contour.

Vitreomacular Traction Syndrome

Key Facts

- Incomplete separation of posterior hyaloid from macula with persistent macular traction causes macular edema and decreased visual acuity
- No sex predilection
- Typically occurs in sixth and seventh decades

Clinical Findings

- Epiretinal membrane (ERM)
- Incomplete posterior vitreous separation with vitreous attachments to macula or optic nerve
- Cystoid macular edema (CME)

Ancillary Testing

- Optical coherence tomography (OCT) is the most useful test, because it accurately images the posterior vitreous hyaloid inserting at the fovea and inducing foveal traction and macular edema
- Fluorescein angiography is typically unnecessary in establishing the diagnosis but has certain characteristics
  - Staining of the optic disc occurs in later frames of the angiogram, and pooling of dye in the foveal cysts may or may not occur

Differential Diagnosis

- ERM
- Postoperative CME
- Central serous retinopathy
- Macular hole

Treatment

- Observation is initially recommended for acute cases because the macular traction will spontaneously resolve in a small percentage of eyes
- Pars plana vitrectomy with manual elevation of the attached posterior hyaloid from the macula
  - Membrane peel should be performed if an ERM is identified either clinically or on OCT

Prognosis

- Untreated vitreomacular traction syndrome tends to cause a slow decline in visual acuity over years from photoreceptor atrophy secondary to chronic CME
- With complete elevation of the posterior hyaloid and peeling of the ERM, most patients gain two or more lines of visual acuity
  - Failure of visual acuity to improve may result from formation of a partial-thickness macular hole at the time of membrane peel or pre-exisiting photoreceptor atrophy

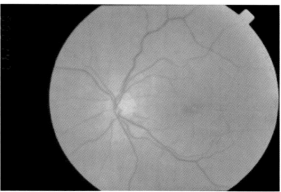

Fig. 9.14 Vitreomacular traction syndrome in a 73-year-old woman with 20/40 visual acuity referred for decreased vision 4 months after successful cataract surgery. A foveal cyst is present on clinical examination.

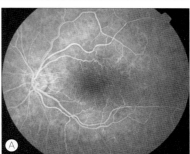

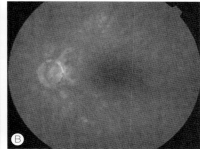

Fig. 9.15 Fluorescein angiography of the same patient as in Fig. 9.14, showing staining of the optic nerve with absent cystoid macular edema in both the (A) middle and (B) late frames of the angiogram.

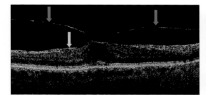

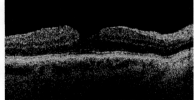

Fig. 9.16 Preoperative OCT identifies the vitreous inserting into the fovea (red arrows) with an overlying epiretinal membrane (yellow arrow) consistent with vitreomacular traction syndrome. The black, hyporeflective spaces in the fovea are intraretinal fluid collections consistent with CME.

Fig. 9.17 One month after pars plana vitrectomy with elevation of the posterior vitreous hyaloid and epiretinal membrane peel, the visual acuity has improved to 20/30 with restoration of a normal foveal contour. One year postoperatively, the visual acuity was 20/25.

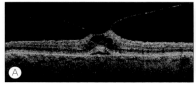

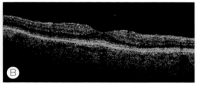

Fig. 9.18 Spontaneous resolution of vitreomacular traction syndrome in a 75-year-old man presenting with 3 weeks of distortion. (A) Vitreomacular traction is present, with elevation of the photoreceptor layer. (B) The vitreous has separated after 1 month of observation, with restoration of a normal foveal contour.

Cystoid Macular Edema

Key Facts

- Accumulation of intraretinal fluid in cystic spaces in the outer plexiform layer of the macula • Occurs from leakage of perifoveal retinal capillaries
- **Multiple etiologies:**
  - ocular surgery (cataract, glaucoma, penetrating keratoplasty, scleral buckle) • laser (panretinal photocoagulation, iridotomy) • uveitis (especially pars planitis) • diabetic retinopathy • radiation retinopathy • acute hypertensive retinopathy • arterial macroaneurysm • central retinal vein occlusion (CRVO) and branch retinal vein occlusion (BRVO) • retinitis pigmentosa • tumors (choroidal hemangioma, retinal capillary hemangioma, choroidal melanoma) • choroidal neovascularization • medication use (topical adrenaline [epinephrine], prostaglandin agonists) • exudative age-related macular degeneration (AMD)

Clinical Findings

- Cystic spaces at the fovea • Dull fovea reflex • Vitritis may be present with active uveitis • Anterior chamber cellular inflammation • Evidence of previous ocular surgery • Intraretinal hemorrhage from branch or central retinal vein occlusion • Hyperemia or swelling of optic nerve

Ancillary Testing

- Fluorescein angiography shows multiple focal areas of leakage, with pooling of dye within cystic spaces in a petaloid pattern
- Cystoid macular edema (CME) is imaged on optical coherence tomography as intraretinal black, hyporeflective spaces
  - Size and number of spaces varies based on CME intensity
- Contact lens examination

Differential Diagnosis

- Juvenile retinoschisis • Goldmann–Favre disease • Nicotinic acid maculopathy • Vitreomacular traction syndrome • Epiretinal membrane (ERM) • Stage 1 macular hole • Solar retinopathy

Treatment

- Treatment based on etiology of CME • Discontinue any topical medications that may exacerbate the condition • Laser photocoagulation in diabetic CME, BRVO, or arterial macroaneurysm • Pars plana vitrectomy with elevation of the posterior hyaloid and/or ERM peel to relieve mechanical retinal traction in ERMs or vitreomacular traction syndrome • In postcataract CME, topical prednisolone acetate 1% combined with a topical non-steroidal anti-inflammatory drug four times daily is the initial course, followed by periocular then intraocular triamcinolone acetonide in recalcitrant cases • Topical, periocular, intravitreal, and oral corticosteroids can be used in sequential order in intermediate or posterior uveitis • Currently, there is no treatment for CRVO, but intravitreal triamcinolone acetonide used off-label may be effective in a small percentage of eyes • Intravitreal anti–vascular endothelial growth factor injections are indicated for exudative AMD

Prognosis

- In postcataract cases after phacoemulsification, angiographic CME occurs in about 10% of healthy eyes 4–12 weeks after surgery and is usually self-limited (Irvine–Gass syndrome) • Clinically significant CME occurs in 0.2–1.4% of cases after phacoemulsification, requiring intervention with topical medications and/or intravitreal corticosteroids • In most cases of pseudophakic CME, patients retain 20/30 or better visual acuity • Visual results in other forms of CME are variable and depend on the underlying etiology

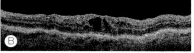

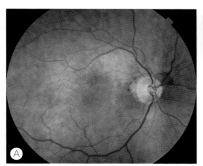

Fig. 9.19 (**A**) Cystic spaces at the fovea are visible in this eye with CME. (**B**) CME is imaged on optical coherence tomography as hyporeflective black spaces located within the retina.

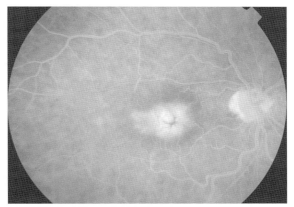

Fig. 9.20 Fluorescein angiography of a different eye from Fig. 9.19, showing cystoid macular edema as petalloid leakage centered at the fovea.

Central Serous Retinopathy

Key Facts

- Idiopathic disorder
- Serous detachment of the neurosensory retina from an area of choroidal leakage
- Area of leakage may be singular or multiple involving one or both eyes
- Most common in men aged 20–50
- Incidence in women increases over age 50
- Occurs mostly in white, Hispanic, and Asian people but is rare in those of African descent
- **Related to:**
  - type A personality • exogenous corticosteroid use • antihistamine use • endogenous hypercortisolism
- **Symptoms include:**
  - metamorphopsia • micropsia • central scotoma • diminished color vision

Clinical Findings

- Decreased visual acuity in the 20/20 to 20/200 range, with most eyes 20/30 or better
- Hyperopic shift is common
- Classic presentation is a round, well-delineated serous retinal detachment in the macula
- Anterior segment, vitreous, optic nerve, and retinal vasculature are normal
- Retinal pigment epithelium (RPE) detachments may be observed
- Chronic central serous retinopathy may lead to atrophy of RPE in macula
- Subretinal tracks of RPE atrophy extending from macula to inferior retina may be seen in eyes with multiple recurrences and previous retinal detachment
- Bullous retinal detachment is an uncommon finding

Ancillary Testing

- Fluorescein angiography elicits pinpoint hyperfluorescence that enlarges with pooling in the neurosensory detachment
  - 20% of eyes will show a classic smokestack pattern
- Multiple areas of leakage are visualized in ≤25% of cases • Indocyanine green angiography shows either a focal area of leakage or larger placoid leaks
- Optical coherence tomography identifies subretinal fluid
  - Chronic cases may have intraretinal cystic changes with or without subretinal fluid

Differential Diagnosis

- Age-related macular degeneration
- Optic nerve pit
- Harada disease
- Choroidal metastasis
- Hypertensive retinopathy
- Retinoschisis
- Lymphoma
- Optic neuritis
- Retinal detachment
- Vitreomacular traction syndrome
- Cystoid macular edema

Treatment

- Observation
- **Laser photocoagulation to areas of focal leakage may speed visual recovery and is reserved for patients with:**
  - symptoms lasting longer than 4 months • bilateral disease • prior episodes that resulted in significant permanent loss of vision • occupational requirements necessitating faster visual recovery
- Photodynamic therapy has been described in select case presentations; however, the long-term efficacy is unknown

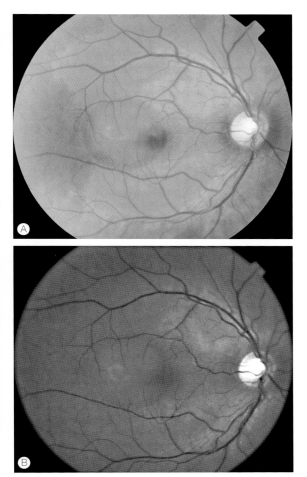

Fig. 9.21 (**A**) Color and (**B**) red-free photographs of a neurosensory detachment of the macula.

Prognosis

- Resolution of neurosensory detachment occurs spontaneously over 3–4 months with observation and 2–3 weeks with laser photocoagulation
- Laser photocoagulation can lead to formation of choroidal neovascularization
- >90% of eyes maintain 20/30 visual acuity or better
- Patients may complain of metamorphopsia, decreased contrast sensitivity, nyctalopia, and dyschromatopsia despite cessation of leakage and resolution of neurosensory detachment • Final visual acuity is not affected whether treatment is by observation or laser
- 20–50% of eyes experience recurrence at 1 year
- 5% of patients will have a complicated clinical course with bullous retinal detachment and RPE degeneration

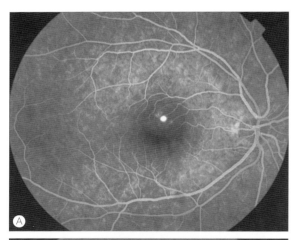

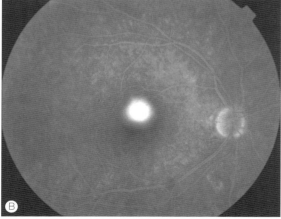

Fig. 9.22 (**A**) Early and (**B**) late frames of a fluorescein angiogram of central serous retinopathy. As the angiogram progresses, there is increasing leakage from the focal spot with progressive pooling of dye into the neurosensory detachment.

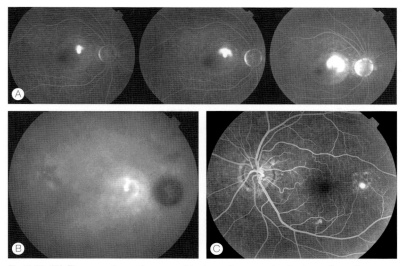

Fig. 9.23 (A) Fluorescein angiogram of leakage in a smokestack configuration. (B) Compared with the fluorescein angiogram, the smokestack pattern of leakage on ICG is not as prominent. (C) Fluorescein angiography of the left eye shows a subclinical focal area of leakage.

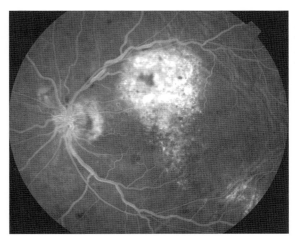

Fig. 9.24 Mottled fluorescence in a flask-shaped configuration on fluorescein angiography of a patient with chronic central serous retinopathy.

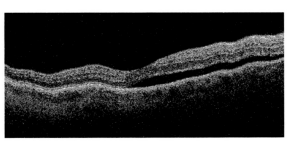

Fig. 9.25 Optical coherence tomography of central serous retinopathy, showing a neurosensory detachment.

Coloboma

Key Facts

- Congenital abnormality
- Failure of the embryonic fissure to close along the inferior portion of the globe that extends from optic nerve to iris
- Variable clinical findings based on extent of embryonic fissure affected
- May be associated with the coloboma, heart defects, choanal atresia, retarded development, genital and ear anomalies (CHARGE syndrome)

Clinical Findings

- Retinochoroidal colobomas are the most common finding, with bare sclera in a staphylomatous cavity inferior to and often involving the optic nerve
- Rhegmatogenous retinal detachment
- Non-rhegmatogenous retinal detachments
- Choroidal neovascularization (CNV) at edge of colobomas
- Inferior notch of the lens secondary to focal absence of zonules
- Inferior iris defect

Ancillary Testing

- Optical coherence tomography (OCT) and fluorescein angiography (FA) are performed if CNV is suspected

Differential Diagnosis

- Morning glory optic disc anomaly
- Congenital tilt of the optic disc
- High myopia with posterior staphyloma

Treatment

- Observation
- Evaluation for heart defects, choanal atresia, retarded development, genital and ear anomalies (CHARGE syndrome) by a primary care physician in infants
- Repair of retinal detachments with pars plana vitrectomy
- Localized retinal detachments centered on optic disc colobomas may be treated with laser demarcation
- Treatment of choroidal neovascularization with intravitreal anti–vascular endothelial growth factor injections

Prognosis

- Vision usually unaffected by the coloboma, except in rare cases in which coloboma extends into macula
- Can be a factor in intraocular lens calculations for cataract surgery

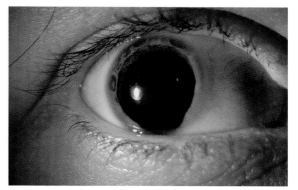

Fig. 9.26 An iris coloboma with a notch in the inferior iris. The pupil is pharmacologically dilated.

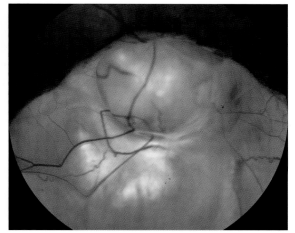

Fig. 9.27 Coloboma of the retina and optic nerve with a prominent staphyloma.

Hydroxychloroquine (Plaquenil) Toxicity

Key Facts

- Medically used in treatment of various connective tissue disorders
- Lower risk of retinal toxicity than chloroquine
- Hydroxychloroquine is well tolerated and rarely causes retinal toxicity in a cumulative dose of <6.5 mg/kg per day
- Incidence of toxicity is very low within first 5 years of treatment
  - Patients with toxicity may be asymptomatic or note central or paracentral scotomas

Clinical Findings

- Macula may be normal even when a scotoma is present
- Pigmentary changes at perifovea
- Loss of foveal reflex
- Macular atrophy in a bull's-eye pattern
- Chronic exposure may lead to a retinitis pigmentatosa–type presentation

Ancillary Testing

- Color vision
- Amsler grid evaluating for metamorphopsia
- 10–2 visual field using a white test spot to evaluate for central or paracentral scotoma
- Multifocal electroretinogram evaluating macular function may detect drug toxicity before overt clinical signs present
- Ultra high-resolution optical coherence tomography more accurately images the photoreceptor layer and may identify photoreceptor loss before clinical evidence of toxicity is visible
- Fluorescein angiography will show window defect in areas of retinal pigment epithelium atrophy

Differential Diagnosis

- Cone dystrophy
- Age-related macular degeneration
- Stargardt disease

Treatment

- Routine yearly retinal examinations to evaluate for toxicity during long-term use
  - When patients have used the medication for >10 years, more frequent examinations every 6 months should be considered
- Discontinue drug if signs of toxicity present on testing or clinical examination

Prognosis

- Toxic effects of the drug may persist even after discontinuation

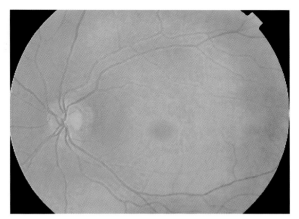

Fig. 9.28 Atrophy of the retinal pigment epithelium surrounding the fovea in a bull's eye pattern from Plaquenil toxicity.

Juvenile X-linked Retinoschisis

Key Facts

- Bilateral
- Rare
- Occurs only in males
- Variable penetrance among affected family members
- Splitting of the nerve fiber layer
- Clinical signs recognized in early childhood
- Mutation of the XLRS1 gene on Xp22
- No known systemic associations

Clinical Findings

- Cystic foveal changes in stellate or spoke-like configuration in nearly all eyes
- Macular pigmentary changes with atrophy in adults
- Peripheral retinoschisis (50% of patients)
- Vitreous hemorrhage (40% of eyes)
- Rhegmatogenous retinal detachment (20% of eyes)
- Exudative retinal detachment
- Demarcation lines from previous retinal detachments
- Macular fold and dragging
- Hypermetropia
- Strabismus
- Amblyopia
- Cataract

Ancillary Testing

- Examine other family members
- No late leakage into foveal cysts on fluorescein angiography
- Electroretinogram with diminished b wave
- Diffuse cystic changes typically throughout entire macula on optical coherence tomography
- Absolute scotoma in areas of peripheral retinoschisis on visual filed examination

Differential Diagnosis

- Retinopathy of prematurity
- Familial exudative vitreoretinopathy
- Retinitis pigmentosa
- Goldmann–Favre disease

Treatment

- Observation
- Pars plana vitrectomy for non-clearing vitreous hemorrhage, especially in children <8–10 years of age at risk for amblyopia
- Repair of retinal detachment with vitrectomy or scleral buckle
- Genetic counseling

Prognosis

- No available treatment for retinal schisis
- Progressive loss of macular function over time, starting in childhood
  - Visual acuity declines to a range of 20/200 by sixth and seventh decades

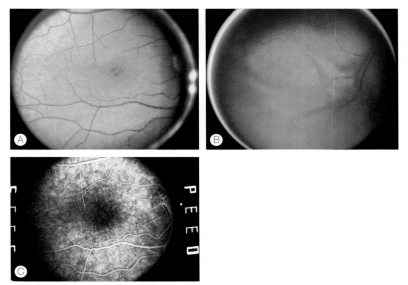

Fig. 9.29 (**A**) Cystic foveal changes in the right eye of a 22-year-old man with juvenile X-linked retinoschisis and 20/40 visual acuity. (**B**) A shallow schisis cavity in the peripheral retina. (**C**) No leakage is present into the foveal cysts during the fluorescein angiogram. On ancillary testing, color vision and the electro-oculogram were normal with an absent b wave on electroretinogram.

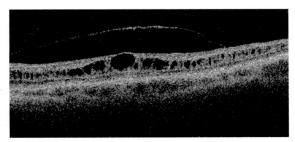

Fig. 9.30 Cystic spaces are present throughout the macula in an eye with juvenile X-linked retinoschisis. A partial separation of the posterior hyaloid is also visible.

Section

10

Retinal Dystrophies

Retinitis Pigmentosa

Key Facts

- Retinal disorder marked by progressive visual loss from photoreceptor death
- Rod–cone dystrophy with rod photoreceptors affected early and cones affected later
- **From most to least common inheritance:**
  - sporadic
  - autosomal dominant
  - autosomal recessive
  - X-linked recessive
- Findings may occur in childhood, with symptoms increasing in second and third decades
- Men affected slightly more than women because of X-linked inheritance pattern
- Night blindness with difficulty adjusting to dim lighting conditions
- Tunnel vision
- Systemic association with Usher, Bardet–Biedl, and Kearns–Sayre syndromes

Clinical Findings

- Typically bilateral and symmetric
- Bone spicule pigmentation or pigment clumping
- Retinal arteriolar narrowing
- Waxy pallor of optic nerve
- Epiretinal membrane
- Atrophy of retinal pigment epithelium (RPE) and choriocapillaris starting in the midperipheral retina and extending with time
- Preservation of RPE in the macula until late in the disease
- Posterior subcapsular cataract
- Cystoid macular edema (CME)
- Carriers will have a normal retina, isolated geographic patches of RPE atrophy and pigment clumping, or diffuse retinal changes
- Rarely symptomatic patients with absent retina findings (retinitis pigmentosa sine pigmento)

Ancillary Testing

- An electroretinogram (ERG) is useful in patients with early disease and minimal clinical findings
  - Early in the disease state, the rod ERG amplitude is affected more than that of the cones
  - With progression of disease, both rod and cone responses are extinguished
- The electro-oculogram (EOG) correlates with the ERG and is reduced
  - An EOG is unnecessary if the ERG is diagnostic
- Farnsworth D-15 color test to evaluate the foveal cone response
  - An abnormal test may predict future central vision loss
- Visual field initially shows a midperipheral ring scotoma, which enlarges peripherally and centrally with disease progression
- Fluorescein angiography (FA) shows areas of choriocapillaris loss
  - Petaloid leakage occurs in CME • In general, FA is not required to make the diagnosis of retinitis pigmentosa
- Optical coherence tomography (OCT) evaluates the presence of epiretinal membrane and CME
  - Ultra high-resolution OCT can document photoreceptor loss

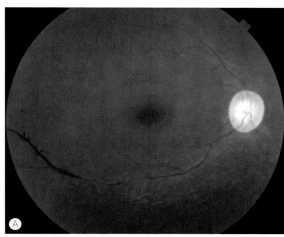

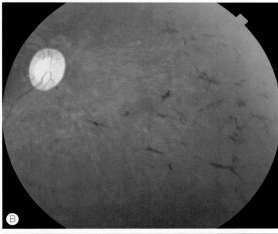

Fig. 10.1 Color photograph of the macula (**A**) and nasal retina (**B**) of the right eye and macula of the left eye (**C**) of a male patient with retinitis pigmentosa. Bone spicule pigmentation is present, with narrowing of the vessels and loss of the RPE outside the vascular arcade.

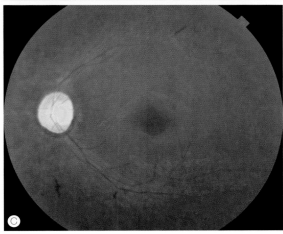

- Medical evaluation should be performed if an associated systemic condition is present

Differential Diagnosis

- Choroideremia
- Congenital stationary night blindness
- Congenital rubella
- Thioridazine retinal toxicity
- Cancer-associated retinopathy

Treatment

- No treatment is effective in halting clinical changes and visual loss
- Vitamin A palmitate 15 000 IU daily has been shown to minimally slow progression of electroretinogram loss
  - Serum liver enzymes should be checked yearly, and treatment should be discontinued if patient falls pregnant
- Acetazolamide 250–500 mg daily for CME
  - Treatment should be continued for 2 months to identify a therapeutic benefit
  - If effective, acetazolamide may need to be continued indefinitely
  - If no response, treatment should be discontinued
- Intravitreal triamcinolone acetonide (4 mg) for refractory CME has been reported, with limited success
- Genetic counseling

Prognosis

- Visual acuity may remain 20/20 even with visual field constriction in typical forms of retinitis pigmentosa
  - Later deterioration of central acuity occurs as cone photoreceptors degenerate
- Patients with X-linked inheritance pattern may have earlier and more pronounced central visual loss because cones are affected earlier in the disease
- Progressive visual loss and night blindness occurs as photoreceptors degenerate

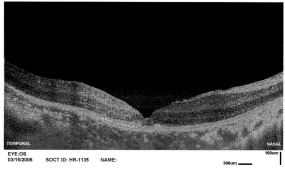

EYE:OS
03/15/2006   SOCT ID: HR-1135   NAME: 100um
    300um ____

Fig. 10.2 A patient with RP imaged with ultra high-resolution OCT, showing loss of the photoreceptor layer and thinning of the retina.

Stargardt Disease (Fundus Flavimaculata)

Key Facts

- Most common inherited macular dystrophy
- Accounts for nearly 7% of all retinal dystrophies
- Inherited primarily as autosomal recessive
- No racial predilection
- Estimated to occur in 1 in 60 000 people
- Stargardt disease and fundus flavimaculata represent different clinical presentations of the same disease
  - Stargardt disease has an onset in first or second decade, with macular atrophy predominating and few flecks
  - Fundus flavimaculata presents in third and fourth decades, with prominent subretinal flecks throughout the retina and less macular atrophy
  - In advanced stages, the clinical picture of the two entities overlaps
- Mutation of the ABCA4 gene

Clinical Findings

- Decreased visual acuity
- Yellow-white subretinal flecks that are round, linear, or pisciform (fish-like) and fluctuate in number over time
- Flecks reabsorb over time and are replaced by atrophy
- Subtle retinal pigment epithelium (RPE) changes with loss of foveal reflex in early stages of disease
- Beaten bronze appearance to macula
- Macular atrophy in advanced chronic disease
- Peripheral degenerative changes
- Vascular attenuation
- Optic disc pallor

Ancillary Testing

- Hypofluorescence of the choroid (known as a dark choroid) visualized on fluorescein angiography in about 85% of eyes, due to accumulation of lipofuscin-like material in RPE
  - Lack of a dark choroid does not rule out Stargardt disease
  - Yellow flecks block fluorescence from lipofuscin accumulation and are hypofluorescent
  - Areas of atrophy transmit fluorescence and are hyperfluorescent
  - In advanced atrophy with destruction of the choriocapillaris, window defect is absent with visualization of the choroidal circulation
- Photopic and scotopic responses on electroretinogram are normal early in the disease process but deteriorate depending on the extent of retinal damage
- Delayed dark adaptation
- Electro-oculogram results (Arden ratio) may show mild abnormalities with advanced disease
- Visual fields show central scotoma correlating to macular atrophy
  - Peripheral fields normal unless peripheral atrophy present

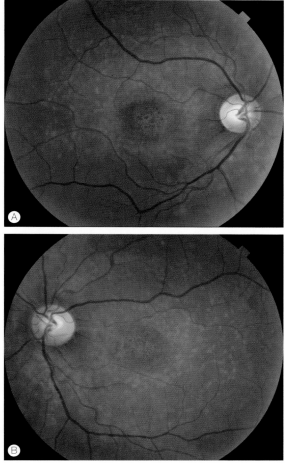

Fig. 10.3 Pisciform flecks and early foveal changes in the (**A**) right and (**B**) left eye of this male patient with Stargardt disease.

Stargardt Disease (Fundus Flavimaculata) (Continued)

Differential Diagnosis

- Cone dystrophy
- Vitelliform macular dystrophy
- Fundus albipunctata
- Retinitis punctata albescens
- Pattern dystrophy
- Ceroid lipofuscinosis
- Familial drusen
- Drug toxicities (e.g. hydroxychloroquine, Plaquenil)
- Best's disease

Treatment

- Low vision evaluation
- No treatment currently exists

Prognosis

- Continued disease progression, with visual acuity declining to 20/200

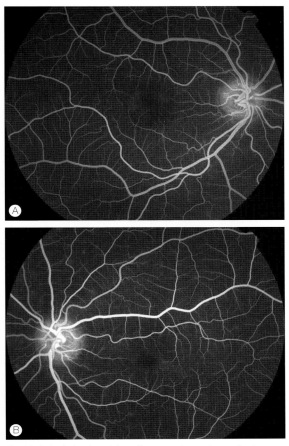

Fig. 10.4 A dark choroid on fluorescein angiography in both the (**A**) right and (**B**) left eye of the same patient from Fig. 10.3.

Cone Dystrophy

Key Facts

- Abnormality of cone function
- Inherited as autosomal dominant, recessive, or X-linked recessive
- Variable disease progression
- Bilateral and symmetric clinical findings
- Common symptoms include difficulty with bright lights (hemeralopia) and decreased visual acuity
- Onset typically occurs in early childhood but may present in middle adulthood

Clinical Findings

- Pigment granularity in the macula early in disease course
- Bull's-eye pattern late in disease
- Temporal disc pallor (rare)
- Tapetal sheen to retina similar to that seen in Oguchi disease (rare)

Ancillary Tests

- Central scotoma present on visual field testing
- Color vision reduced
- The photopic electroretinogram (ERG) and photopic flicker ERG are abnormal, the scotopic ERG normal
  - If rod function loss is present, it is very mild and not to the point of a cone–rod dystrophy as seen in retinitis pigmentosa
- Fluorescein angiography shows a mottled hyperfluorescence early in the disease course
  - As a bull's-eye pattern evolves clinically, the classic ring of hyperfluorescence surrounding a residual island of hypofluorescence is present
- Examine other family members for evidence of similar clinical findings

Differential Diagnosis

- Stargardt disease
- Chloroquine toxicity

Treatment

- None available

Prognosis

- Visual loss is progressive to 20/200 or worse in both eyes
- Patients with earlier onset of disease typically have a more severe form

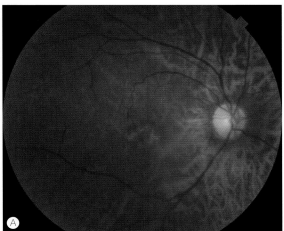

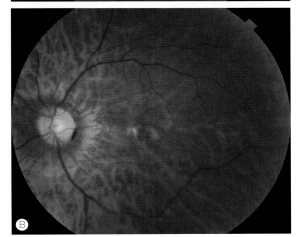

Fig. 10.5 The (**A**) right and (**B**) left eye of a male patient with a bull's-eye maculopathy. Note the ring of retinal pigment epithelium atrophy surrounding a small island of more normal appearing retina. ERG showed diminished scotopic responses.

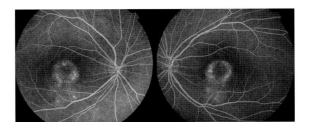

Fig. 10.6 Fluorescein angiography of a different patient from Fig. 10.5, with a cone dystrophy showing a ring of hyperfluorescence around an area of relative hypofluorescence consistent with a bull's-eye pattern.

Best Disease

Key Facts

- Rare disorder
- Autosomal dominant with variable penetrance
- Affects all races equally
- Variable clinical expression and age of onset among family members
- Accumulation of lipofuscin-like material in retinal pigment epithelium (RPE) cells
- No systemic associations

Clinical Findings

- Yellow, well-demarcated, egg yolk–like vitelliform lesion in the macula (classic appearance)
- Pseudohypopyon occasionally occurs from layering of the yellow material in the macula
- Focal areas of RPE hyperplasia in the macula
- Pattern dystrophy–like markings
- Mulitfocal vitelliform lesions throughout posterior pole (multifocal Best disease)
- Choroidal neovascularization (CNV)
- Atrophy and scarring of the macula in eyes with resolved vitelliform lesions

Ancillary Tests

- Blockage of fluorescence occurs with the classic yolk-like lesion
  - Linear hyperpigmentation occurring over time also creates blockage of fluorescence, creating a pattern dystrophy–like appearance
  - Window defect present in areas where the vitelliform lesion has thinned or RPE atrophy is present
  - Active leakage occurs when CNV present
- Electroretinogram normal
- Electro-oculogram is abnormal with an Arden ratio of <1.5
- Genetic counseling

Differential Diagnosis

- Pattern dystrophy
- Stargardt disease
- Adult onset vitelliform dystrophy
- Age-related macular dystrophy

Treatment

- No treatment for the vitelliform lesions is available
- Treatment of CNV with anti–vascular endothelial growth factor intravitreal injections may be beneficial; however, no reports regarding this form of treatment have been published
- Examine all family members

Prognosis

- Variable visual outcome, but acuity may remain 20/40 or better
- **Lesions evolve over time:**
  - becoming scrambled
  - resolving completely
  - becoming fibrotic scars
  - forming new clumps of yellow material with RPE hyperplasia similar to pattern dystrophies

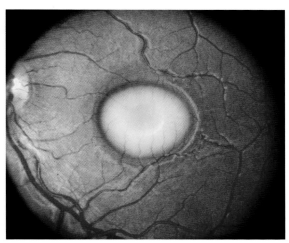

Fig. 10.7 Best disease with a yolk-like vitelliform lesion in the macula.

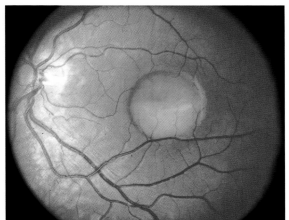

Fig. 10.8 Pseudohypopyon in an eye with Best's disease.

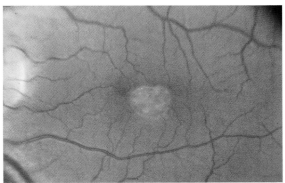

Fig. 10.9 The macular lesion in this eye with Best's disease and 20/70 visual acuity shows early fibrosis with loss of the yolk-like appearance.

Pattern Dystrophy

Key Facts

- Various gray-, yellow-, or orange-pigmented patterns occurring in the macula
- Usually bilateral and symmetric
- Typically inherited as autosomal dominant with variable expressivity among family members
- Most patients are asymptomatic or have very mild visual disturbances
- Lesions typically present clinically within the fourth to sixth decades

Clinical Findings

- Irregular pigmentary deposits in the macula in a variety of patterns
- Granular appearance to retinal pigment epithelium
- Choroidal neovascularization (CNV)

Ancillary tests

- Fluorescein angiography more clearly delineates the macular changes compared with clinical examination, because the pigmented areas block fluorescence
  - Angiography is also useful in identifying areas of CNV, which leak when clinically active
- Electroretinogram typically normal
- Electro-oculogram (EOG) results are variable
  - If all family members have an abnormal EOG, Best's disease must be considered

Differential Diagnosis

- Age-related macular degeneration
- Drusen
- Best disease
- Stargardt disease

Treatment

- Observation
- Anti–vascular endothelial growth factor therapy should be considered when CNV is diagnosed; however, its efficacy is unknown

Prognosis

- Visual acuity is usually unaffected unless CNV occurs
- Late in the disease course macular atrophy may occur, leading to a mild decline in visual acuity

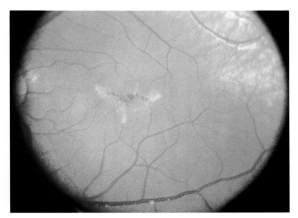

Fig. 10.10 Butterfly-shaped pattern dystrophy.

Choroideremia

Key Facts
- Bilateral
- X-linked recessive
- Most common hereditary choroidal dystrophy
- Occurs in first and second decades
- Nyctalopia

Clinical Findings
- Early in the disease course, retinal findings in the midperiphery can have a salt and pepper appearance or be similar to early retinitis pigmentosa with bone spicule pigmentation
- Choroidal atrophy starts at the equator and spreads both peripherally and centrally
- Atrophy of choroidal vessels
- Sparing of retinal vessels, with a normal caliber and appearance
- Optic nerve maintains normal appearance
- Macula is spared until late in the disease course as the disease progresses from the midperiphery to the peripheral retina and macula

Ancillary Tests
- Peripheral visual field loss that becomes more prominent with disease progression
- Electroretinogram (ERG) shows abnormal rod and cone responses early in the disease course even when the clinical picture is mild
  - Carriers have a normal ERG
- Prominent atrophy of choriocapillaris on fluorescein angiography
- Genetic counseling

Differential Diagnosis
- Generalized choroidal dystrophy
- Retinitis pigmentosa (advanced)
- Gyrate atrophy
- Rubella
- Syphilis
- Thioridazine

Treatment
- None available

Prognosis
- Central visual acuity maintained usually until the fourth decade, when atrophy wipes out the fovea, leading to visual acuity <20/200 in most patients
- Female carriers typically maintain normal visual acuity given the X-linked recessive inheritance

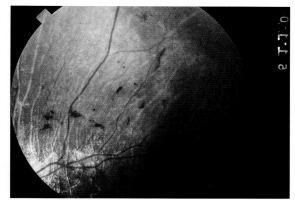

Fig. 10.11 Peripheral atrophy with bone spicule pigmentation at the midequator in a patient with choroideremia.

Gyrate Atrophy

Key Facts

- Very rare generalized choroidal dystrophy
- Autosomal recessive
- Bilateral
- Early symptoms include nyctalopia and peripheral visual field loss
- Abnormality of ornithine aminotransferase

Clinical Findings

- Well-circumscribed, scalloped appearing areas of chorioretinal atrophy with hyperpigmented borders surrounded by normal retina in the midperiphery
- Over time the lesions will coalesce
- Posterior pole often appears normal

Ancillary Tests

- Electroretinogram markedly diminished with abnormalities of both photopic and scotopic response
- Visual fields are constricted even with minimal peripheral retinal involvement
- Elevated plasma ornithine levels
- Fluorescein angiography shows loss of choriocapillaris in affected retina
- Genetic counseling

Differential Diagnosis

- Choroideremia
- Uveitis
- Retinitis pigmentosa

Treatment

- Vitamin B_6 increases ornithine aminotransferase activity and reduces ornithine levels
- Reduce arginine in the diet because it is a precursor of ornithine

Prognosis

- Lowering plasma ornithine levels has mixed results on slowing progression of disease
- Most patients have a visual acuity of <20/200 starting in the fourth decade

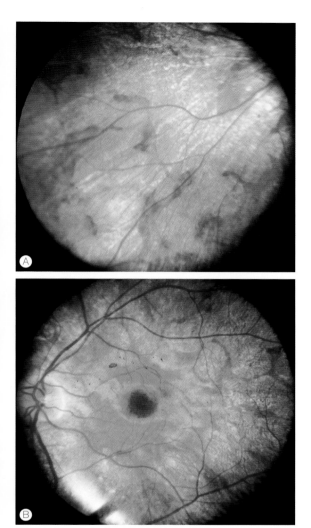

Fig. 10.12 (**A**) Well-demarcated scalloped areas of chorioretinal atrophy that are primarily in the peripheral retina, with (**B**) involvement of the macula.

Central Areolar Choroidal Dystrophy

Key Facts
- Autosomal dominant
- Rare condition
- Onset in second decade

Clinical Findings
- Solitary, well-circumscribed circular area of chorioretinal atrophy in the macula that is bilateral and symmetric
- Early granularity of the fovea progressing to complete central atrophy
- Hyperpigmentation at the border of normal and abnormal retina

Ancillary Tests
- Fluorescein angiography shows absence of the choriocapillaris, with transmission hyperfluorescence late in the angiogram
- Electroretinogram normal, indicating that this is a macular and not a global retinal disorder
- Electro-oculogram normal
- Color vision decreased in advanced cases

Differential Diagnosis
- Age-related macular degeneration
- Myopic degeneration
- Stargardt disease
- Cone dystrophy
- North Carolina macular dystrophy
- Best's disease

Treatment
- Observation

Prognosis
- Early in the disease, visual acuity is excellent but progressively declines to 20/400 as chorioretinal atrophy progresses

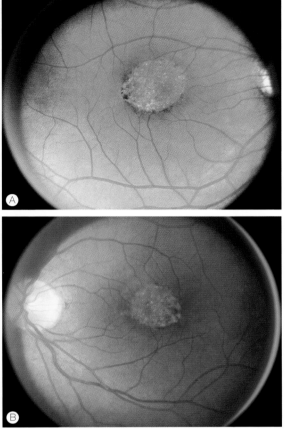

Fig. 10.13 A well-circumscribed area of chorioretinal atrophy bilaterally in a patient with central areolar choroidal dystrophy.

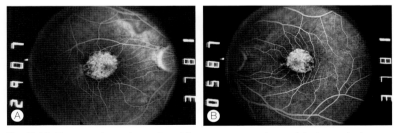

Fig. 10.14 Fluorescein angiography of the same eyes shows late transmission fluorescence in the macula.

Fundus Albipunctatus

Key Facts

- Form of congenital stationary night blindness
- Non-progressive loss of night vision present since birth
- Autosomal recessive
- Rod abnormality (scotopic response) with normal cone response (photopic)
- Etiology unknown
- Caused by delay in regeneration of rod and cone pigment

Clinical Findings

- Round, punctate, discrete white spots in a regular pattern that tend to remain unchanged over time
- Occurs in the posterior pole out to midperiphery
- Mild granular pigmentary changes in the macula may occur

Ancillary Testing

- The white spots are historically not associated with any fluorescein abnormalities; however, focal areas of fluorescence of spots may be seen with apparent enlargement of the foveal avascular zone
- Reduction of a and b waves occurs on electroretinogram (ERG)
  - With prolonged dark adaptation, there is normalization of the ERG
- Visual fields are normal

Differential Diagnosis

- Retinitis punctata albescens

Treatment

- Observation

Prognosis

- Vision is unaffected
- Night blindness stable and not progressive

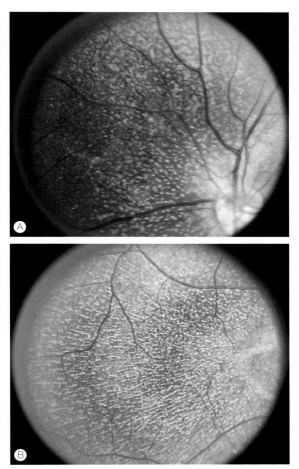

Fig. 10.15 (**A,B**) Color photographs of fundus albipunctatus showing multiple, regularly spaced, punctate, yellow-white spots that radiate out from the optic nerve.

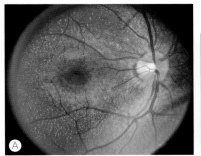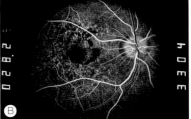

Fig. 10.16 (**A**) Mild pigmentary changes are visible in the fovea. (**B**) Fluorescein angiogram showing patchy blockage of fluorescence in the fovea with staining of the spots.

North Carolina Macular Dystrophy

Key Facts

- Rare form of macular degeneration
- Autosomal dominant
- Originally discovered in a family from North Carolina but occurs worldwide
- Now known as MCDR1 (macular dystrophy, first retinal subtype mapped)
- Clinical findings present at birth

Clinical Findings

- Atrophy of retinal pigment epithelium and choriocapillaris
- Bilateral and symmetric
- Coloboma of the macula
- Choroidal neovascularization (CNV)

Ancillary Testing

- Fluorescein angiography if CNV suspected
- Color photograph for documentation
- Electroretinogram, electro-oculogram, and color vision testing are normal
- Genetic counseling

Differential Diagnosis

- Central areolar choroidal dystrophy
- Age-related macular degeneration
- Toxoplasmosis

Treatment

- Observation
- CNV may be treated with intravitreal anti-vascular endothelial growth factor or photodynamic therapy
  - No formal studies evaluating treatment are available

Prognosis

- Visual acuity is usually better than the clinical picture suggests and can range from 20/20 to 20/200
- CNV will lead to decreased visual acuity in a small subset of patients
- Clinical findings usually do not progress

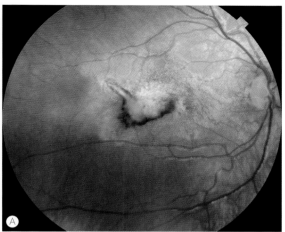

Fig. 10.17 The (**A**) right and (**B**) left eye of a 3-year-old boy with North Carolina macular dystrophy that was originally diagnosed shortly after birth. A fibrotic scar from inactive CNV is present in the right eye.

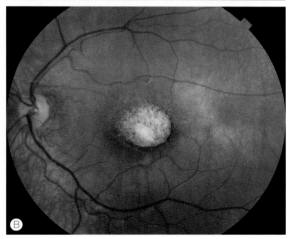

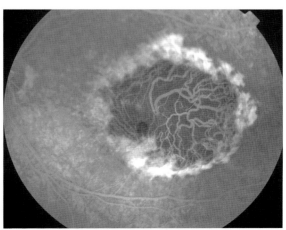

Fig. 10.18 Fluorescein angiography of the father of the patient in Fig. 10.17 shows complete atrophy of the retinal pigment epithelium and choriocapillaris.

Adult Onset Vitelliform Dystrophy

Key Facts

- Form of pattern dystrophy
- Autosomal dominant with variable expressivity
- Occurs within the fourth and sixth decades
- Most patients are asymptomatic, with lesions discovered on routine clinical examination

Clinical Findings

- Solitary, minimally elevated, round, yellow deposit in the fovea
- Bilateral and symmetric
- Foveal lesions are about one-third of disc area
- Central gray clump in the yellow lesion may develop

Ancillary Testing

- Electroretinogram is normal
- Electro-oculogram is normal or slightly reduced
- Optical coherence tomography shows a medium-reflective dome-shaped elevation in the outer retina
- Lesions on fluorescein angiography are hypofluorescent
  - Occasionally a small hyperfluorescent ring around the hypofluorescent central lesion is present

Differential Diagnosis

- Best disease
- Stargardt disease
- Age-related macular degeneration

Treatment

- Observation

Prognosis

- Vision may be normal or slightly diminished in the 20/25 to 20/60 range

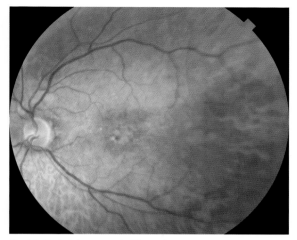

Fig. 10.19 Adult onset vitelliform dystrophy present as a yellow, minimally elevated deposit in the fovea. A mirror image was present in the right eye (not shown).

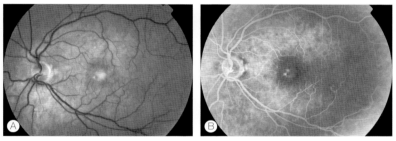

Fig. 10.20 (**A**) Red-free and (**B**) late fluorescein angiogram of the left eye from Fig. 10.19, showing blockage with mild mottled staining of the vitelliform lesion.

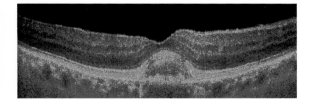

Fig. 10.21 A mound-like elevation of the retinal pigment epithelium and photoreceptor layer is present on ultra high-resolution optical coherence tomography of the eye in Fig. 10.19.

Section

11

White Dot Syndromes

Multiple Evanescent White Dot Syndrome

Key Facts

- Patients present with acute onset of decreased vision, with complaints of photopsias and temporal or paracentral scotoma
- Women affected more commonly than men
- Occurs in healthy persons in the second to fifth decades
- Monocular, but bilateral cases occur
- Etiology unknown
- Viral prodrome present in about 50% of patients

Clinical Findings

- Multiple gray-white, punctate dots at the level of the retinal pigment epithelium in the posterior pole, sparing the fovea
- Granularity of fovea
- Mild iritis and vitritis occasionally identified

Ancillary Testing

- Fluorescein angiography (FA) shows early punctate hyperfluorescence in a wreath-like configuration in the macula, with late staining
- Indocyanine green shows hypofluorescent spots in macula and peripheral retina
  - The hypofluorescent spots are larger than the white dots identified clinically
  - Hypofluorescence may be imaged around optic nerve
- Variable visual field defects identified, with enlarged blind spot the most common
- The visual field loss is greater than what would be expected from the clinical examination and FA
- Abnormalities seen on electroretinogram in acute phase of disease, with normalization when multiple evanescent white dot syndrome resolves

Differential Diagnosis

- Optic neuritis
- Acute posterior multifocal pigmented placoid epitheliopathy
- Birdshot retinochoroidopathy
- Punctate inner choroidopathy
- Multifocal choroiditis
- Toxoplasmosis
- Diffuse unilateral subacute neuroretinitis

Treatment

- Observation, because the disorder is self-limited and spontaneously resolves

Prognosis

- Excellent prognosis, because most eyes improve to 20/30 or better within 2–3 months
- Recurrent disease rarely occurs

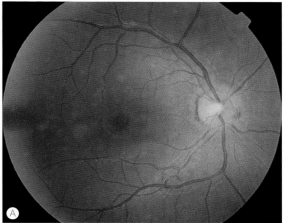

Fig. 11.1 (**A**) Peripheral white dots in the temporal macula in a patient with active multiple evanescent white dot syndrome. (**B**) Four months later, mild foveal granularity is more visible. A few of the spots are still visible temporal to the fovea.

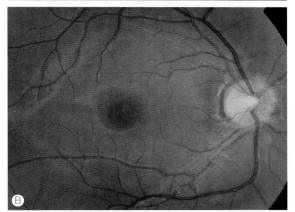

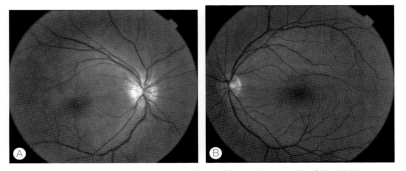

Fig. 11.2 (**A**) Focal spots are visible in this red-free photograph of the right eye. (**B**) The left eye is normal.

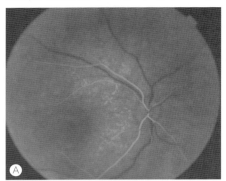

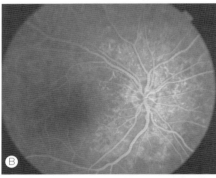

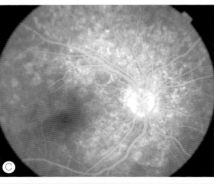

Fig. 11.3 Fluorescein angiogram of the patient in Fig. 11.2 shows hyperfluorescence in a wreath-like pattern around the fovea in the (A) early, (B) mid, and (C) later frame of the angiogram. (D) The fluorescein angiogram of the left eye is normal.

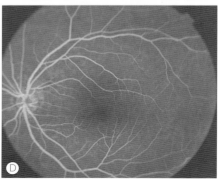

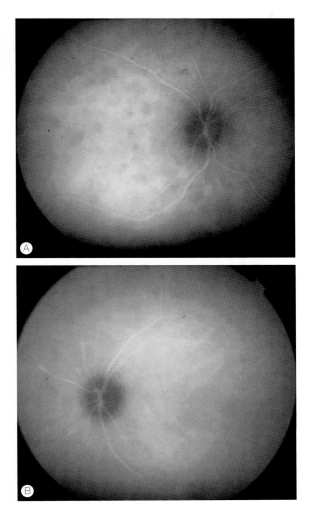

Fig. 11.4 Multiple hypofluorescent spots are visible on indocyanine green in the affected right eye from the patient in Figs 11.2 and 11.3 (**A**) but are absent in the unaffected left eye (**B**).

Multifocal Choroiditis and Panuveitis

Key Facts

- Posterior uveitis of unknown etiology • Chronic disorder with multiple recurrences • Spectrum of white dot disorders along the lines of punctate inner choroidopathy or ocular histoplasmosis syndrome • Women affected more than men • No racial predilection • Presentation with blurred vision, scotoma, floaters, photophobia, or mild ocular discomfort • Myopia
  - Primarily a bilateral disorder

Clinical Findings

- Anterior chamber inflammation (mild to moderate)
- Vitreous inflammation (mild to moderate)
- Acute lesions are yellow-gray and evolve into inactive scars with hyperpigmented edges that are punched out
  - Lesions are focused in macula and nasal periphery and occur isolated in groups or in a linear fashion • Peripapillary lesions may occur similar to those in ocular histoplasmosis syndrome
- Swelling or hyperemia of optic nerve
- Epiretinal membrane
- Cystoid macular edema
- Subretinal fibrosis
- Choroidal neovascularization (most common cause of vision loss)

Ancillary Testing

- Enlarged blind spot on visual field test in ≤50% of patients
  - Other visual field defects occurring less frequently include central, paracentral, and cecocentral scotoma • Peripheral field defects occasionally occur and are unrelated to actual areas of chorioretinal atrophy • Visual fields may also be normal
- Electroretinogram abnormalities vary depending on disease severity
- Active lesions are hyperfluorescent on fluorescein angiography
  - Window defect is present in chronic, inactive lesions

Differential Diagnosis

- Punctate inner choroidopathy • Ocular histoplasmosis syndrome • Sarcoidosis
  - Toxoplasmosis • Birdshot chorioretinopathy

Treatment

- Topical prednisolone acetate 1% for anterior chamber inflammation • Sub-Tenon corticosteroid injections every 2–3 weeks as necessary to control intraocular inflammation • Oral prednisone starting with 60–80 mg daily, followed by a slow taper based on clinical response
- Intravitreal anti–vascular endothelial growth factor should be considered for CNV, especially when subfoveal
  - Laser photocoagulation may be considered for juxtafoveal and extrafoveal CNV

Prognosis

- Up to 66% of all eyes achieve 20/40 or better visual acuity • Decreased vision of 20/200 or worse occurs from formation of CNV, cystoid macular edema, or extensive macular scarring (20–30% of eyes) • Initial presenting visual acuity is not a predictor of final visual outcome • Cataract and glaucoma secondary to corticosteroid use can cause visual loss and should be treated appropriately

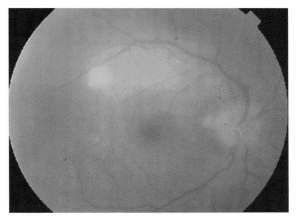

Fig. 11.5 Color photograph of the right eye, showing disc edema and a hazy view of retinal details from active vitritis.

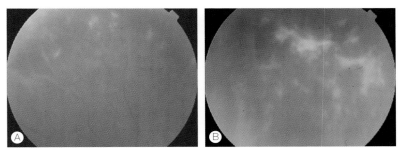

Fig. 11.6 (**A**) Peripheral color photograph of the right eye in Fig. 11.5, showing yellow-gray lesions consistent with active choroiditis. (**B**) The active lesions are irregular in shape and variable in size.

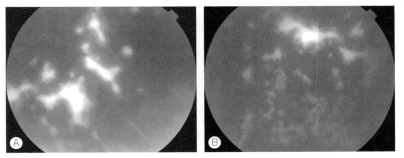

Fig. 11.7 The active lesions are hyperfluorescent on fluorescein angiography. (**A,B**) Window defect is present peripheral to the active lesions, representing previous inflammatory lesions that are now chronic and inactive (**B**).

Punctate Inner Choroidopathy

Key Facts
- Occurs in healthy young myopic women
- Bilateral
- Unknown etiology

Clinical Findings
- Absent vitreous inflammation
- Yellow-white lesions at level of inner choroid
- Most lesions are in the macula, with occasional lesions in midperiphery and nasal to optic nerve
- Choroidal neovascularization (CNV) may occur in active lesions or from the edge of chronic scars
- Chronic lesions show atrophy with pigmentation
- Acute lesions may heal with bridging fibrosis to other lesions

Ancillary Testing
- On fluorescein angiography, acute lesions hyperfluoresce early and leak late
  - Chronic scars show staining
  - If CNV present, there is more prominent fluorescence with late leakage
- Visual field testing may show enlargement of the blind spot out of proportion to the number of lesions
  - Other findings include central or paracentral scotoma
- Electroretinogram usually normal
- Optical coherence tomography useful in following subretinal fluid collections when active CNV present
- Laboratory tests not beneficial

Differential Diagnosis
- Ocular histoplasmosis syndrome
- Myopic degeneration
- Multifocal choroiditis and panuveitis
- Acute multifocal posterior placoid pigment epitheliopathy

Treatment
- Observation, because most cases are self-limited
- When CNV present, treatment options include:
  - Oral corticosteroids
  - Laser photocoagulation to CNV outside the fovea
  - Photodynamic therapy
  - Intravitreal anti–vascular endothelial growth factor

Prognosis
- Visual prognosis depends on presence of CNV
  - Most patients have 20/40 or better acuity, with 20/200 or worse acuity occurring with subfoveal CNV
- No prospective randomized trials evaluating efficacy of treating subfoveal CNV exist

SECTION 11 • White Dot Syndromes

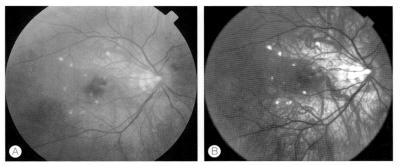

Fig. 11.8 (**A**) Color photograph of yellow-white punctate lesions focused in the macula. At the fovea, there is subretinal hemorrhage around a pigmented lesion. (**B**) Red-free photograph accentuates the focal spots in the macula.

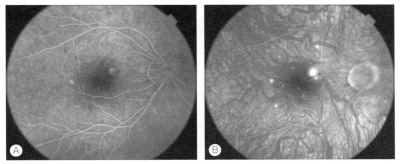

Fig. 11.9 Hypefluorescence of the active lesions in the (**A**) middle and (**B**) late phase of the angiogram of the eye in Fig. 11.8. The juxtafoveal hyperfluorescence nasal to the fovea represents CNV. Note that the active punctate inner choroidopathy lesions are more fluorescent in the later phase of the angiogram.

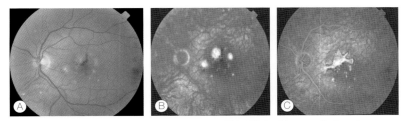

Fig. 11.10 Punctate inner choroidopathy and CNV (**A**) in this myopic female patient who shows coalescence of the active lesions from beseline (**B**) and at 1-month (**C**).

Acute Posterior Multifocal Placoid Pigment Epitheliopathy

Key Facts

- Uncommon inflammatory syndrome of posterior pole
- Unknown etiology
- Typically develops between the third and sixth decades
- No racial predilection
- No gender predilection
- Cause of sudden, rapid vision loss
- May be associated with cerebral vasculitis
- Usually bilateral

Clinical Findings

- Acute lesions are well-defined, irregularly shaped yellow-white placoid lesions located primarily in the macula at the level of the retinal pigment epithelium and choroid
- Lesions vary in number and size and may become confluent
- Healing of lesions occurs within days to weeks of initial presentation
  - Lesions fade and become mottled with pigmentation and atrophy
- Absence of vitreous inflammation

Ancillary Testing

- Fluorescein angiography of acute lesions shows early choroidal hypofluorescence followed by late hyperfluorescence
  - Chronic lesions show mottled staining
  - Angiography often identifies lesions of varying age on presentation
- Indocyanine green (ICG) angiography of acute lesions shows choroidal hypofluorescence in early and late frames of the angiogram
  - Chronic lesions on ICG are also hypofluorescent but not as extensive as the acute lesions

Differential Diagnosis

- Multiple evanescent white dot syndrome
- Serpiginous choroiditis
- Vogt–Koyanagi–Harada syndrome
- Punctate inner choroidopathy
- Multifocal choroiditis
- Birdshot retinochoroiditis
- Viral or bacterial chorioretinitis
- Metastatic tumors

Treatment

- No definitive treatment exists
- Observation, because most cases resolve spontaneously
- If neurologic symptoms present, a short course of oral prednisone may be instituted because a link to cerebral vasculitis has been identified
- Some ophthalmologists advocate the use of prednisone for all acute cases; however, no benefit has ever been identified

Prognosis

- Usually a self-limited disease, with visual acuity improving to 20/40 or better in most cases within 2–6 weeks
- Decreased visual acuity associated with macular scar formation or atrophy

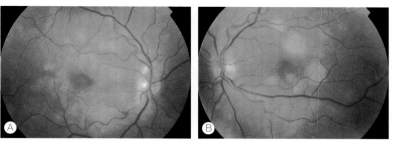

Fig. 11.11 Creamy yellow-white lesions at the level of the RPE in an acute case of acute posterior multifocal placoid pigment epitheliopathy. Despite the acute nature, pigmentation is present at the edge of the more chronic lesions (**A,B**).

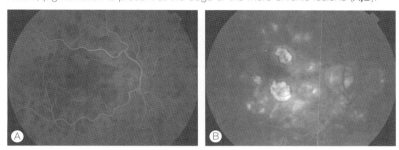

Fig. 11.12 The lesions are hypofluorescent in the early phases of the angiogram (**A**) and hyperfluorescent in the later phases (**B**). The more chronic lesions as seen in the color photograph in Fig. 11.11 show staining with a hypofluorescent halo.

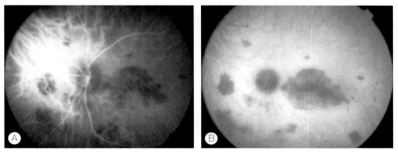

Fig. 11.13 Hypofluorescence of the lesions in both the (**A**) early and (**B**) late frame of the ICG.

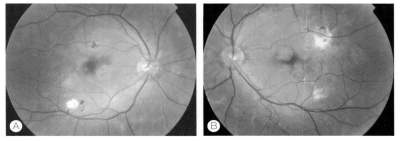

Fig. 11.14 Four years after an acute bout of acute posterior multifocal placoid pigment epitheliopathy, circular areas of chorioretinal scars and scattered subretinal fibrosis are visible in both the (**A**) right and (**B**) left eye of this young male patient.

Serpiginous Choroiditis

Key Facts

- Rare, chronic, progressive disorder marked by alternating periods of quiescence followed by reactivation of the disease • At presentation, most patients show evidence of previous active disease • No sexual predilection • Unknown etiology but presumed to be inflammatory • Occurs in young or middle-aged adults • Usually no associated systemic disease • Presents with decreased vision or scotoma

Clinical Findings

- Active disease presents as creamy yellow lesions at the level of the retinal pigment epithelium (RPE) and choroid in a serpiginous and geographic configuration typically extending from the optic disc • Disease is less commonly centered in the macula (macular serpiginous), sparing the peripapillary region • Inactive disease marked by chorioretinal atrophy with mottling of the RPE • Recurrent disease occurs at the leading edge of inactive disease and spreads in a contiguous fashion • Choroidal neovascularization (CNV) rarely occurs at the edge of chorioretinal atrophy • Mild vitritis may occur during active disease

Ancillary Testing

- Hypofluorescence of active lesions occurs in the early phases of fluorescein angiography (FA), with staining of the edges of the lesion in the late phases
  - Staining occurs in chronic, inactive lesions
- Indocyanine green is similar to FA, with hypofluorescence of the active lesion in early and later phases and hyperfluorescence at the lesion edge in later phases
  - Hypofluorescence tends to be more extensive than the clinically present lesions
  - Staining occurs in chronic lesions
- Visual fields delineate scotoma from the disease but are not useful in diagnosis or treatment
- Electroretinogram and electro-oculogram normal

Differential Diagnosis

- Acute posterior multifocal pigmented placoid epitheliopathy • Toxoplasmosis • Ocular histoplasmosis syndrome • Tuberculosis • Syphilis • Sarcoidosis • Posterior scleritis • Best disease • Lymphoma • Metastatic tumor • Choroidal osteoma • Central areolar choroidal dystrophy

Treatment

- Oral corticosteroids (1 mg/kg per day) are the most common treatment for acute lesions • Cyclosporin A • Combination therapy with corticosteroids, cyclosporin A, and azathioprine • Interferon alfa-2a • Laser photocoagulation for extrafoveal CNV • Intravitreal anti-VEGF for subfoveal CNV

Prognosis

- Poor visual acuity when active disease affects the fovea • Because of the rare nature of the disease, no randomized prospective trials have been performed to elucidate the most effective means of treatment

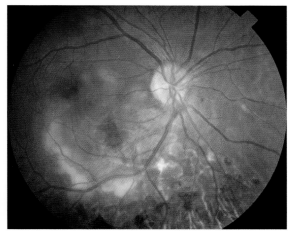

Fig. 11.15 In this eye with serpiginous chorioretinitis, active chorioretinitis is present as a creamy yellow lesion extending toward the fovea adjacent to chorioretinal scar.

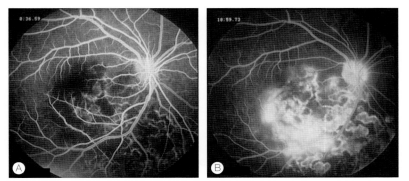

Fig. 11.16 FA of the patient in Fig. 11.15 shows early hypofluorescence of areas of active chorioretinitis in the arteriovenous phase (**A**), with late leakage of these same active areas in later frames of the angiogram (**B**). Staining occurs at the edges of the inactive chorioretinal scars.

Birdshot Retinochoroidopathy

Key Facts

- Rare form of bilateral posterior inflammation
- Chronic remitting and relapsing disorder
- Unknown etiology
- Genetic association with HLA-A29
- No obvious sexual preference
- Onset in fourth to seventh decade, with a median age of onset of 50 years
- Caucasians primarily affected
- Commonly presents with floaters

Clinical Findings

- Anterior chamber inflammation
- Vitreous inflammation
- Absence of snow banking, as seen in intermediate uveitis
- Multiple creamy yellow-orange spots at the level of the choroid or retinal pigment epithelium
  - The lesions are bilateral and symmetric and appear to radiate from the optic nerve in a linear fashion • The lesions are concentrated at the equator, with sparing of the macula
- Hypopigmentation of the macula may occur late in the disease • Cystoid macular edema (CME)
- Choroidal neovascularization

Ancillary Testing

- When the classic lesions are identified, diagnostic testing is unnecessary
  - More mildly affected eyes in which the diagnosis is not obvious may require blood work that includes complete blood count with differential, syphilis serology, Lyme titers, chest x-ray for tuberculosis and sarcoidosis, and angiotensin converting enzyme or serum lysozyme for sarcoidosis
- Blood work to identify HLA-A29, because ≥90% of all patients with birdshot chorioretinopathy carry this HLA marker
- Fluorescein angiography shows disc staining and vascular leakage
  - The lesions do not transmit choroidal fluorescence and show mild fluorescence only in the late frames of the angiogram • The hypopigmented lesions are more obvious clinically than angiographically
- Electroretinogram (ERG) is variable and depends on length and severity of disease
  - In most eyes with disease, there is a subnormal rod and cone response
    - 30-Hz flicker is the most sensitive measure for retinal dysfunction • ERG may be abnormal even with mild or absent disease, so ERG may be useful for observing patients

Differential Diagnosis

- Intermediate uveitis (pars planitis)
- Harada disease
- Sympathetic ophthalmia
- Acute posterior multifocal placoid pigment epitheliopathy
- Serpiginous choroidopathy
- Multiple evanescent white dot syndrome
- Ocular histoplasmosis syndrome
- Intraocular lymphoma

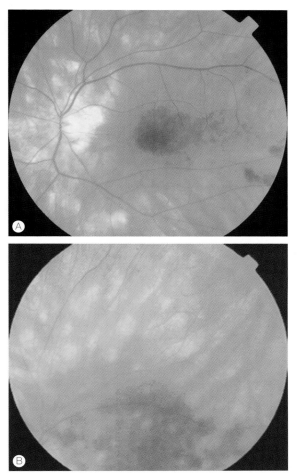

Fig. 11.17 (**A**) Color photograph of the left posterior pole, showing hypopigmented spots consistent with birdshot retinochoroidopathy. (**B**) The spots radiate outward from the vascular arcade.

Birdshot Retinochoroidopathy (Continued)

Treatment

- Oral corticosteroids • Intravitreal corticosteroids • Sub-Tenon's corticosteroids
- Non-corticosteroid immunosuppressive agents (cyclosporine, azathioprine, methotrexate)

Prognosis

- Visual prognosis varies and depends on length and severity of disease
  - The disease is progressive and usually leads to slow visual decline
- Data supporting long-term treatment efficacy with immunosuppressive agents is limited
  - Early use of immunosuppressive agents may limit the formation of CME
- Both CME and retinal degeneration will lead to visual field loss and decrease in visual acuity

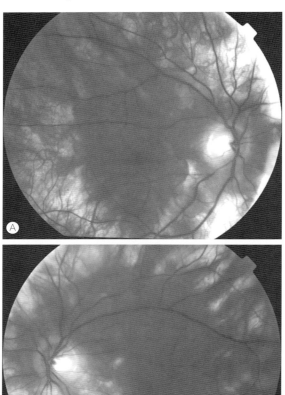

Fig. 11.18 The hypopigmented spots are more prominent on red-free photographs of the (**A**) right and (**B**) left eye.

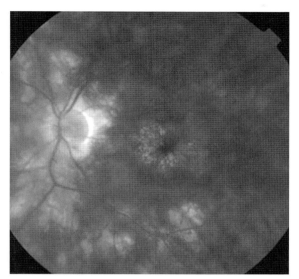

Fig. 11.19 Fluorescein angiogram of the eye in Fig. 11.17, with a petalloid pattern of leakage consistent with cystoid macular edema.

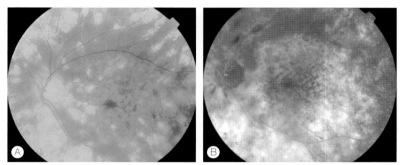

Fig. 11.20 (A) Color photograph and (B) fluorescein angiography of a patient with advanced birdshot retinochoroidopathy. Prominent hypopigmented spots are noted on the color photograph inside the vascular arcade. Retinal pigment epithelial atrophy is present in the macula, leading to the window defect seen on the angiogram.

Ocular Histoplasmosis Syndrome

Key Facts

- Caused by fungus *Histoplasma capsulatum*
- Endemic to the Mississippi and Ohio River valleys
- Vision loss occurs primarily from subfoveal choroidal neovascularization (CNV)
- Men and women are equally affected
- Ocular findings may be unilateral or bilateral
- Up to 5% of patients with a positive skin test for *H. capsulatum* have peripheral retinal scars

Clinical Findings

- Normal or decreased visual acuity
- Punched-out chorioretinal spots in midperiphery and macula
- Peripapillary atrophy
- Linear scars in midperipheral retina
- CNV with associated hemorrhage and subretinal fluid
- Absence of vitreous inflammation
- Submacular scar from previous CNV

Ancillary Testing

- Fluorescein angiography (FA) to evaluate for presence and location of CNV
- Indocyanine green angiography to evaluate for CNV when blockage from blood prevents accurate diagnosis of CNV with FA
- Optical coherence tomography (OCT) to scan for presence of CNV, as well as for presence of intraretinal and subretinal fluid
  - OCT is useful in following fluid collections to determine the success of treatment and whether retreatment is necessary
- Histoplasmin skin test positive in 95% of patients with clinical retinal findings; however, skin testing is not recommended because it may cause reactivation of inactive chorioretinal scars

Differential Diagnosis

- Age-related macular degeneration
- Punctate inner choroidopathy
- Multifocal choroiditis
- Myopic degeneration
- Acute multifocal posterior placoid epitheliopathy
- Sarcoid uveitis

Treatment

- Laser photocoagulation to juxtafoveal and extrafoveal CNV
- Photodynamic therapy with verteporfin for subfoveal CNV
- Intravitreal anti-vascular endothelial growth factor (VEGF)
- Submacular surgery only as a final option when laser or intravitreal anti-VEGF injections are ineffective

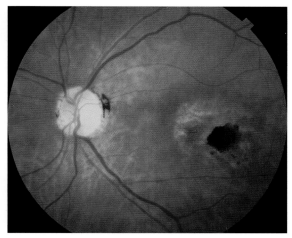

Fig. 11.21 Peripapillary atrophy and a pigmented macular scar with surrounding atrophy from previous subfoveal CNV in an eye with ocular histoplasmosis syndrome. The visual acuity measures counting fingers.

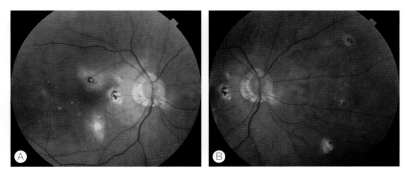

Fig. 11.22 (A) Ocular histoplasmosis with multiple perifoveal scars and 20/20 visual acuity. (B) Peripapillary atrophy and peripheral punched out chorioretinal scars are present.

Prognosis

- Excellent prognosis for patients without macular scars or for those who do not develop subfoveal CNV
- Eyes without macular scars are at very low risk of developing CNV
- The Macular Photocoagulation Study showed a reduction in severe visual loss at 5 years from 44% in observed eyes with extrafoveal CNV to 9% in eyes treated with argon laser photocoagulation
  - In eyes with juxtafoveal CNV, the MPS showed at 5 years that 28% of eyes had severe vision loss in the untreated group compared with 12% in the photocoagulation group
- Treatment of subfoveal CNV with photodynamic therapy using verteporfin resulted in a median increase in visual acuity from baseline of 1.2 lines or six letters (Verteporfin in Ocular Histoplasmosis Study Group)
- There is no proven benefit to submacular surgery for subfoveal CNV compared with observation (Submacular Surgery Trial)

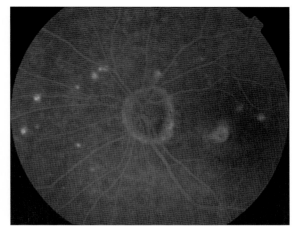

Fig. 11.23 Fluorescein leakage from a subfoveal CNV, with staining of peripapillary atrophy and peripheral retinal scars in the left eye.

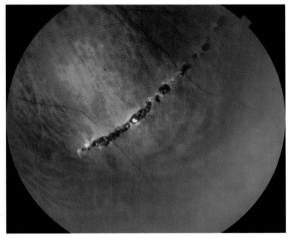

Fig. 11.24 Peripheral linear pigmentation in an eye with ocular histoplasmosis syndrome.

Section

12

Inflammatory Diseases

Posterior Scleritis

Key Facts

- Rare inflammatory disorder of the sclera occurring posterior to equator
  - Unilateral • Women affected more than men • Associated with an underlying systemic disorder in about 50% of patients (rheumatoid arthritis most common) • May present with decreasing vision and severe, deep eye pain

Clinical Findings

- In pure posterior scleritis, the anterior segment may be normal • Dilated episcleral vessels with edematous sclera when the anterior sclera is involved • Iritis • Choroiditis • Localized choroidal mass • Elevated IOP • Ciliary body detachment causing a shallow anterior chamber and angle closure glaucoma • Exudative retinal detachment • Chorioretinal folds • Optic disc edema

Ancillary Testing

- **Laboratory testing should include:**
  - an evaluation of syphilis with rapid plasma reagin or fluorescent treponemal antibody absorption test • rheumatoid factor and antinuclear antibody for systemic connective tissue disorder • chest x-ray and purified protein derivative to evaluate for tuberculosis • angiotensin-converting enzyme level and chest x-ray in sarcoidosis • C-ANCA for Wegener granulomatosis
- Ultrasound of the posterior segment to evaluate for a thickened sclera and the T sign
  - The T sign is due to fluid, imaged as a dark hyporeflective signal, collecting in the sub-Tenon's space perpendicular to the hyporeflective signal of the optic nerve • The T sign is not present in every case
- Fluorescein angiography shows either punctate hyperfluorescence in macula or a focal plaque of hyperfluorescence
  - Alternating light and dark band from chorioretinal folds may be imaged
- CT with contrast may delineate the sclera (ring sign)

Differential Diagnosis

- Vogt–Koyanagi–Harada syndrome • Amelanotic choroidal melanoma

Treatment

- Topical prednisolone acetate 1% when anterior uveitis present
- Oral prednisone (1 mg/kg per day) required in severe cases of posterior scleritis, followed by a slow taper over ≥4–6 weeks
- Intravenous methylprednisolone 500 mg to 1 g in very severe cases
- Other immunomodulating agents may be required in cases that are unresponsive to prednisone
  - Administration of these drugs should be in conjunction with a rheumatologist

Prognosis

- Most cases of posterior scleritis and associated clinical findings resolve, with improvement in visual acuity, after administration of oral prednisone

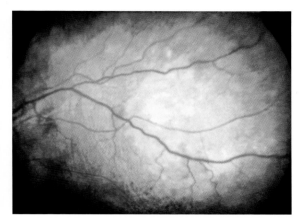

Fig. 12.1 Posterior scleritis presenting as a focal area of inflammation in the macula.

Vogt–Koyanagi–Harada Syndrome

Key Facts

- Bilateral panuveitis of unknown etiology • Presents with decreased vision • Occurs in third to fifth decades but also seen in early childhood • More common in darkly pigmented individuals of Asian or American Indian descent • Inflammation is targeted at pigmented cells in uvea, central nervous system (CNS), and skin
- **CNS manifestations include:**
  - tinnitus • hearing loss • stiff neck • ataxia • focal neurologic deficits
- Cutaneous changes in skin, hair, and lashes are delayed findings • Viral prodrome may occur

Clinical Findings

- Exudative retinal detachment may be extensive, multifocal, or localized to peripapillary and macular region • Mild or absent vitreous inflammation • Punctate yellow-white lesions at level of retinal pigment epithelium • Hyperemia or swelling of optic nerve • Retinal striae • Vascular tortuosity • Sunset glow fundus may occur from depigmentation after resolution of neurosensory detachment • Pigmentary changes • Subretinal fibrosis • Choroidal neovascularization • Anterior uveitis • Angle closure glaucoma from ciliary body swelling • Open angle glaucoma from chronic inflammation • Poliosis • Vitiligo • Madarosis • Alopecia

Ancillary Testing

- Multiple punctate areas of early, intense hyperfluorescence in areas of exudative retinal detachment, with pooling of dye in the later phases, occur on fluorescein angiography • Multiple focal areas of leakage are identified on indocyanine green • A neurosensory detachment is visible on optical coherence tomography
- Thickening of the choroid with low reflectivity occurs on B-mode ultrasound
  - Exudative retinal detachments will also be visualized on ultrasound
- Pleocytosis present on lumbar puncture; this is unnecessary for diagnosis or treatment

Differential Diagnosis

- Sympathetic ophthalmia • Hypertensive retinopathy • Posterior scleritis • Idiopathic uveal effusion syndrome • Metastatic carcinoma • Central serous chorioretinopathy

Treatment

- Oral prednisone starting at 1 mg/kg followed by a slow taper over months for treatment of posterior uveitis and neurosensory detachments • Cyclosporine 5–10 mg/kg has been used in refractory cases • Topical prednisolone acetate 1% for anterior uveitis

Prognosis

- Rapid visual acuity improvement to 20/40 or better can occur in two-thirds of patients or more with aggressive early corticosteroid treatment

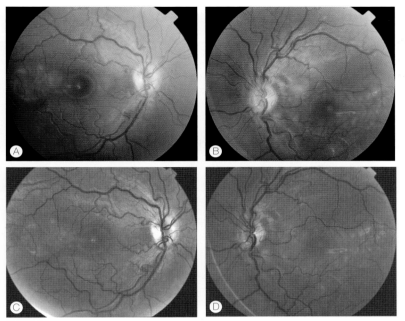

Fig. 12.2 Color and red-free photographs of the (**A,C**) right and (**B,D**) left eye of a 12-year-old boy on presentation for decreased visual acuity. Well-circumscribed neurosensory detachments are visible in the macula, with yellow-white spots present at the level of the retinal pigment epithelium. Vascular tortuosity is present in both eyes.

Vogt–Koyanagi–Harada Syndrome (Continued)

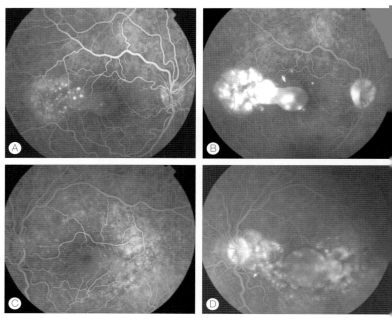

Fig. 12.3 Punctate hyperfluorescence combined with late pooling of dye into the neurosensory detachment is present in both the (**A,B**) right and (**C,D**) left eye on fluorescein angiography. Late staining of the optic disc occurs in both eyes in the late phases of the angiogram (B,D).

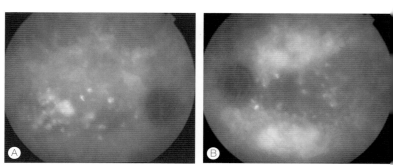

Fig. 12.4 Multiple foci of hyperfluorescence occurring within the neurosensory detachment on indocyanine green. Note in the left eye on ICG (**B**) there is a relative hypofluorescence from the neurosensory detachment with fluorescence along the superior and inferior temporal arcades not seen on the FA in Fig. 12.3B,D.

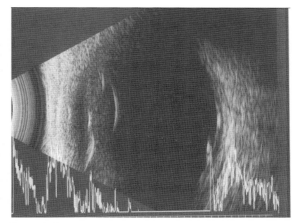

Fig. 12.5 B-mode ultrasound with low reflectivity and thickening of the choroid.

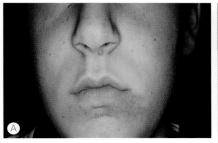

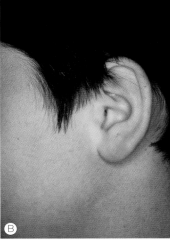

Fig. 12.6 (**A**) Vitiligo and alopecia above the left upper lip and (**B**) vitiligo of the preauricular area occurring 2 years after the initial ocular findings.

Behçet Disease

Key Facts

- Systemic inflammatory disorder associated with chronic, recurrent uveitis
- Unknown etiology
- Primarily bilateral
- Men more severely affected than women
- Occurs in third to fifth decades of life
- 50 times more prevalent in Japan than in North America or Europe
- Triad of uveitis, oral ulcers, and genital ulcers
- Considered an autoimmune disease, with antibodies to mucous membranes identified in 50% of cases

Clinical Findings

- Anterior chamber cells
- Hypopyon (the hallmark of Behçet disease but quite rare)
- Vitreous cells
- Retinal hemorrhage
- Sheathing of retinal veins
- Arterial and venous occlusions
- Cystoid macular edema
- Oral aphthous ulcers
- Genital ulcers
- **Skin findings include:**
  - folliculitis • erythema nodosum • acne-like exanthem • vasculitis (rare)
- Arthritis of knees and ankles that is not deforming

Ancillary Testing

- HLA-B5 levels may be elevated in patients from eastern Mediterranean countries and Japan
- Laboratory testing to rule out other causes of uveitis

Differential Diagnosis

- Systemic lupus erythematosus
- Sarcoidosis
- Syphilis

Treatment

- Topical prednisolone acetate 1% hourly to treat anterior chamber inflammation
- Periocular corticosteroid injection with triamcinolone acetonide 40 mg
- Systemic prednisone 1 mg/kg daily
- Intravitreal triamcinolone acetonide 4 mg in eyes when cystoid macular edema is present that does not respond to periocular or systemic steroids
- Immunosuppressive agents (cyclosporin A or azathioprine) when prolonged systemic prednisone alone is not effective or prolonged treatment is required
- Rheumatologic consultation

Prognosis

- Because of the vascular occlusive component, visual prognosis may be poor
- Chronic uveitis that may last for years

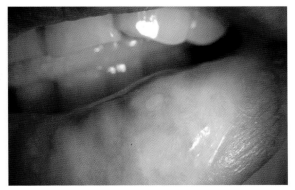

Fig. 12.7 Oral aphthous ulcer in a female patient with active Behçet disease.

Section

13

Infectious Diseases

Progressive Outer Retinal Necrosis

Key Facts

- Patients are typically infected with HIV
- The CD4 count is usually <100/mm^3
- Caused by varicella-zoster virus (VZV)
- May be proceeded by dermatomal zoster
- Incidence is declining with the use of highly active antiretroviral therapy
- Starts as a unilateral disease, but rapidly affects both eyes

Clinical Findings

- Minimal or absent intraocular inflammation
- Starts as deep, white, multiple areas of retinal opacification in the periphery or macula
- Opacified areas become confluent, eventually affecting the entire retina
- Rapid spread of disease over days
- No vasculitis
- Absence of hemorrhage
- Sparing of venules
- Optic atrophy late in disease course
- Pigment mottling in previously infected retina
- Rhegmatogenous retinal detachment

Ancillary Testing

- PCR testing of intraocular fluid for VZV
  - This is usually not necessary—the clinical picture is usually diagnostic

Differential Diagnosis

- Acute retinal necrosis
- Cytomegalovirus retinitis

Treatment

- Acyclovir, ganciclovir, and foscarnet alone or as combination intravenous therapy
- Intravitreal foscarnet (2.4 mg/0.1 mL) every 3 days
- Laser photocoagulation encircling the macula to prevent posterior progression of retinal detachment
- Pars plana vitrectomy with endolaser and silicone oil tamponade for retinal detachment

Prognosis

- Untreated the disease rapidly progresses, leading to blindness within weeks
- Antiviral therapy intravenously or intravitreally alone or as combination treatments is rarely effective but may protect the contralateral eye from disease formation
- Retinal detachments occur in the vast majority of patients

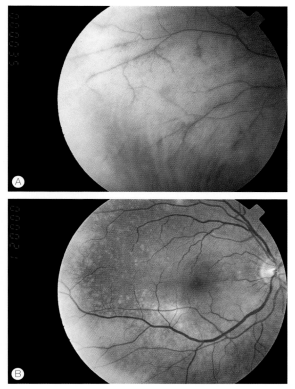

Fig. 13.1 Deep, white areas of retinitis in the peripheral retina of a patient with HIV. (a) There is sparing of the venules and a clear view without vitritis. (b) The retinitis extends to the edge of the macula, with punctate satellite lesions.

Acute Retinal Necrosis

Key Facts

- Viral infection of the retina
- Etiology is herpesvirus infection typically from herpes simplex virus (HSV) or varicella-zoster virus (VZV); rarely cytomegalovirus (CMV)
- Rare
- No sexual or racial predilection
- Patients usually have a normal immune system
- May be unilateral or bilateral

Clinical Findings

- White, opaque retinitis that starts at in the peripheral retina as small patches, rapidly spreads circumferentially (becoming confluent), and then moves toward the macula
- Vitritis that may be dense and limit views to the retina
- Anterior chamber inflammation with keratic precipitates
- Retinal vasculitis primarily affecting the arterioles
- Occlusive vasculopathy
- Optic neuropathy
- Pigment mottling in previously infected retina
- Scleritis
- Rhegmatogenous retinal detachment

Ancillary Testing

- PCR analysis of intraocular fluid for the evaluation of HSV and VZV
- Fluorescein angiography is usually not employed but may delineate areas of ischemia from occlusive vasculopathy

Differential Diagnosis

- Progressive outer retinal necrosis
- Cytomegalovirus retinitis
- Syphilis
- Behçet disease

Treatment

- Intravenous acyclovir 1500 mg/m^2 per day in three divided doses for 7–10 days
- Prednisone 40–60 mg daily 2 days after initiation of acyclovir to reduce intraocular inflammation
- Aspirin 650 mg daily to treat thrombotic occlusion of the choroidal and retinal vessels
- Prophylactic peripheral laser at the edge of affected and normal retina may be considered to prevent retinal detachment of the macula
- Pars plana vitrectomy with silicone oil tamponade for rhegmatogenous retinal detachment

Prognosis

- If untreated, blindness will occur from either optic neuropathy or retinal detachment

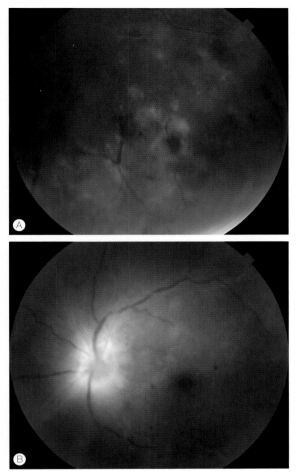

Fig. 13.2 (**A**) A 33-year-old man presented with anterior uveitis, scleritis, vitritis, and circumferential, patchy retinitis. Intraretinal hemorrhages and vasculitis were present. (**B**) The macula is hazy from the vitritis, and disc edema and satellite infiltrates are noted just outside the vascular arcade.

Cytomegalovirus Retinitis

Key Facts

- Slowly progressive herpes virus affecting the retina • Full-thickness retinal necrosis • Retinitis occurs in immunocompromised patients when the CD4 count is <50 cells/mm^3 • No sexual or racial predilection • Unilateral or bilateral • With the introduction of highly active antiretroviral therapy (HAART), the incidence of cytomegalovirus (CMV) retinitis has dramatically decreased
  • Patients may be asymptomatic or complain of decreased vision, floaters, or visual field defects

Clinical Findings

- Early infection may appear as a white lesion similar to a cotton wool spot occurring anywhere within the retina alone or as multiple foci • Retinitis slowly spreads in a brushfire-like pattern, with a leading edge of active retinitis (retinal whitening) and intraretinal hemorrhage • Pigmentation and atrophy remain in areas of inactive retinitis • Papillitis • Vascular sheathing • Mild or absent vitritis
  • Rhegmatogenous retinal detachment from multiple small holes in affected retina

Ancillary Testing

- HIV test • CD4 count • Color photographs of affected retina to compare with older pictures to determine if subtle reactivation is present • PCR testing of aqueous or vitreous samples or retinal biopsy when the diagnosis is in doubt (these techniques are rarely used)

Differential Diagnosis

- Progressive outer retinal necrosis • Acute retinal necrosis • Toxoplasmosis

Treatment

- HAART includes one or more viral protease inhibitors and two or more reverse transcriptase inhibitors
  • This treatment should be instituted immediately in untreated patients
- In CMV retinitis that threatens the macula or in patients already receiving HAART, treatment with intravitreal or intravenous medications below should be instituted promptly
- **Ganciclovir:**
  • intravenous ganciclovir 5 mg/kg twice daily for 2 weeks as an induction, followed by 5 mg/kg daily as maintenance therapy; the main systemic side effect is neutropenia • oral ganciclovir 600 mg five times daily as maintenance therapy • intravitreal ganciclovir 200 μg/0.1 mL once or twice weekly • ganciclovir implant releases 1 μg/h for 6–12 months
- **Foscarnet:**
  • intravenous foscarnet as an induction dose of 60 mg/kg three times daily or 90 mg/kg twice daily for 2 weeks, followed by a maintenance dose of 90–120 mg/kg daily; nephrotoxicity is the main side effect and is offset with adequate intravenous hydration • intravitreal foscarnet 2400 μg/0.1 mL once or twice weekly
- **Cidofovir (intravenous):**
  • intravenous cidofovir 5 mg/kg weekly for 2 weeks as maintenance dose, followed by 5 mg/kg every 2 weeks as maintenance; side effects include nephrotoxicity (offset with intravenous fluids) • intravitreal cidofovir should be avoided because of the uveitis and hypotony that may form
- Valganciclovir is an oral prodrug of ganciclovir with 10 times the bioavailability and is administered in a dose of 900 mg/day
- Pars plana vitrectomy with silicone oil for rhegmatogenous retinal detachments

Prognosis

- Left untreated, CMV retinitis carries a high risk of permanent vision loss from macular involvement and/or rhegmatogenous retinal detachment
- Treatment with HAART induces immune system recovery
  • With the implementation of HAART therapy in the 1990s, the incidence of CMV retinitis has dramatically decreased to levels at which the infection is rarely seen

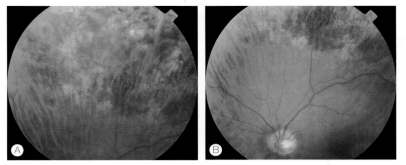

Fig. 13.3 Active CMV retinitis presenting as retinal whitening and hemorrhage in the superior retina outside of the macula.

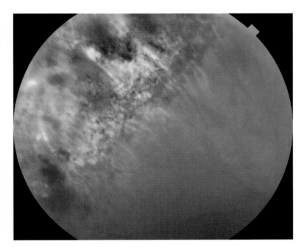

Fig. 13.4 The inactive CMV retinitis in this HIV-positive female patient shows chorioretinal scarring with pigmentation.

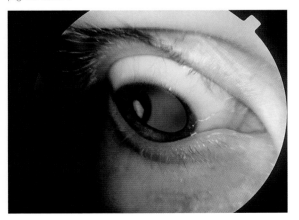

Fig. 13.5 A ganciclovir implant visible through a dilated pupil.

Toxoplasmosis Retinochoroiditis

Key Facts

- Most common form of posterior uveitis
- Caused by infection with *Toxoplasma gondii*
- Cats are definitive hosts and oocytes are excreted in feces
- Spread to humans via ingestion of contaminated soil or meat (acquired) or maternal–fetal transmission in previously uninfected women (congenital)
- Healthy humans inactivate *T. gondii* organisms, which then lie dormant in the retina until reactivation occurs
- Cases are either congenital or acquired
- Serologic evidence of systemic infection can increase with age
- Retinochoroiditis occurs most often in second and third decades
- Usually unilateral
- Occurs more often in areas with poor sanitation, increased consumption of raw meat, and temperate climate

Clinical Findings

- Anterior uveitis
- Vitritis that may be dense ('headlight in the fog')
- Single or multiple areas of chorioretinitis
- Reactivation of chorioretinitis occurs adjacent to a chorioretinal scar
- Macular scar in congenital toxoplasmosis
- Vascular sheathing
- Retinal hemorrhage
- Vitreous contraction with posterior vitreous detachment
- Vitreous strands
- Papillitis
- Optic neuritis
- Retinal detachment

Ancillary Testing

- IgG and IgM *Toxoplasma* antibodies
- PCR of aqueous
- CT or MRI in immunocompromised patients with active ocular toxoplasmosis to evaluate for central nervous system involvement

Differential Diagnosis

- Syphilis
- Sarcoidosis
- Tuberculosis
- Cytomegalovirus
- Acute retinal necrosis

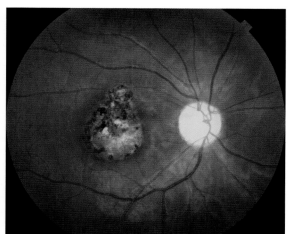

Fig. 13.6 Macular scar in a patient with congenital toxoplasmosis.

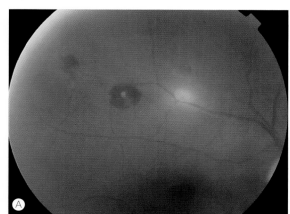

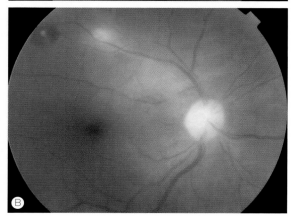

Fig. 13.7 A focal area of chorioretinitis secondary to toxoplasmosis, with an adjacent chorioretinal scar, is present along the superior temporal arcade (**A,B**). The view is hazy from active vitritis.

Treatment

- Topical prednisolone acetate 1% with a cycloplegic agent when anterior uveitis is present
- Observation when lesions are peripheral and do not threaten vision
- Antibiotics should be considered when chorioretinitis involves the optic nerve or macula
  - Pyrimethamine, sulfadiazine, and folinic acid is the historical antibiotic treatment of choice, but this combination is rarely used today
  - More commonly, trimethoprim-sulfamethoxazole or azithromycin therapy is initiated
  - Antibiotic treatment should be used for 6 weeks; however, no study has ever shown that antibiotic coverage is beneficial
- Oral prednisolone is used when macular edema or optic neuritis is present, with treatment initiated 2 days after starting antibiotics
- Immunocompromised patients require antibiotics

Prognosis

- In immunocompetent patients, the disease is usually benign and self-limited

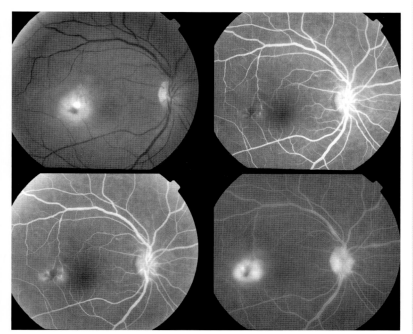

Fig. 13.8 A focal area of hyperfluorescence is present in the macula from active toxoplasmosis chorioretinitis on this fluorescein angiogram. Notice the slight staining of the veins around the optic nerve, as well as staining of the optic disc.

Cataract Surgery–associated Endophthalmitis

Key Facts

- Severe intraocular infection after cataract surgery
- Acute postoperative endophthalmitis occurs within 6 weeks of intraocular surgery
- Incidence <0.1% after phacoemulsification surgery but may have increased recently because of the adoption of sutureless temporal clear corneal incisions
  - In acute cases, *Staphylococcus epidermidis* (coagulase-negative staphylococci) is the most common pathogen; *Staph. aureus*, *Streptococcus* species, and gram-negative organisms are less common
- Chronic cases occur >6 weeks after surgery, are usually more indolent, and are commonly caused by *Propionibacterium acnes*, *Staph. epidermidis*, and *Corynebacterium* species
- Offending organisms usually originate on the lid and conjunctival surface
- Risk factors include active blepharitis, conjunctivitis, dacryocystitis, or the use of contaminated eyedrops
- Operative risk factors include poor preparation and draping technique, vitreous loss, contaminated equipment, and sutureless corneal wounds
- No racial or sexual predilection

Clinical Findings

- Acute decline in visual acuity
- Pain
- Lid edema
- Conjunctival injection
- Anterior chamber inflammation
- Fibrin in anterior chamber
- Hypopyon
- Vitreous inflammation
- Intraretinal hemorrhage
- White intracapsular plaque from *P. acnes* (chronic)

Ancillary Testing

- Ultrasound when vitreous inflammation blocks visualization of the retina
- Anterior chamber and vitreous samples are sent for cultures to identify the offending microorganism
  - If *P. acnes* suspected, anaerobic cultures should be obtained and grown for a minimum of 2 weeks

Differential Diagnosis

- Phacoanaphylactic uveitis
- Normal postoperative inflammation

Treatment

- Based on the Endophthalmitis Vitrectomy Study (EVS), anterior chamber and vitreous tap followed by intravitreal antibiotics (vancomycin 1 mg/0.1 mL and ceftazidime 2.25 mg/0.1 mL) are indicated when visual acuity is hand motion or better
  - Pars plana vitrectomy followed by intravitreal antibiotics is performed when visual acuity measures light perception
- Retreatment with intravitreal antibiotics is rarely required and is performed only if the clinical infection does not clear—in these cases, ocular pain often persists

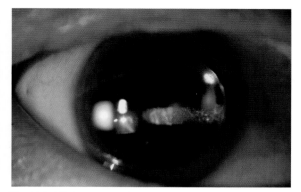

Fig. 13.9 Mild postoperative endophthalmitis is present in slit-lamp beam as only mild anterior vitreous inflammation without a hypopyon. Visual acuity measured 20/30, with a complaint of a decline in vision 1 week postoperatively. Antibiotics were injected into the vitreous, with a return of vision to 20/20.

- Intravitreal dexamethasone (400 μg/0.1 mL) may be beneficial and is often injected into the vitreous in acute cases in addition to intravitreal antibiotics, but its efficacy has not been evaluated in a clinical trial
- Topical broad-spectrum antibiotics ranging from four times daily to hourly based on the treating physician's preference
- Prednisolone acetate 1% every 1–2 h to treat intraocular inflammation
- Systemic antibiotics may be used but no benefit has been identified in clinical trials
- *P. acnes* may be difficult to treat, eventually requiring vitrectomy with removal of the lens capsule and intraocular lens if infection persists

Prognosis

- *Staph. epidermidis* has the best prognosis, with 60% of eyes achieving 20/40 or better vision
  - *Staph. aureus, Streptococcus species*, and gram-negative organisms have a poorer prognosis
- Regardless of treatment, at 9–12 months 53% of eyes had visual acuity ≥20/40, 74% ≥ 20/100, and 15% < 5/200
  - 5% of patients had no light perception
- In eyes with light perception vision, immediate vitrectomy and intravitreal antibiotics compared with intravitreal injections alone produced better final visual acuity in the ≥20/40 group (33% versus 11%) and ≥20/100 group (56% versus 30%), and fewer patients with severe vision loss (20% versus 47%)
- In eyes with hand motion visual acuity or better, vitrectomy offers no advantage over injection of antibiotics alone
- Following injection of antibiotics into the vitreous cavity, the amount of intraocular inflammation temporarily increases over 24 h, followed by a slow clearing of residual inflammatory cells over a period of weeks to months
  - Vitrectomy surgery is rarely required to clear residual vitreous debris

Non–cataract Surgery-related Endophthalmitis

Key Facts

- Severe intraocular infection • Can be classified as traumatic, bleb-related, or endogenous • Endophthalmitis associated with penetrating keratoplasty and pars plana vitrectomy rarely occurs • *Streptococcus pneumoniae* and *Haemophilus influenzae* are the most common organisms causing bleb-associated endophthalmitis and may occur years after surgery • Traumatic endophthalmitis occurs more frequently in rural settings, with *Bacillus* species and *Staphylococcus epidermidis* the most common offending agents, occurring within days to weeks after injury
- **Endogenous endophthalmitis usually affects:**
  - patients who have wound infections, urinary tract infections, and indwelling catheters • patients with diabetes • the immunocompromised • patients who use intravenous drugs

Clinical Findings

- Anterior chamber and vitreous inflammation • Hypopyon • Conjunctival injection and chemosis • Lid edema and erythema • White, milky bleb • Bleb leak • Corneal edema • Fibrin in the anterior chamber • Retinal hemorrhages • Retinal infiltrates (Candida infection) • Intraocular foreign body (IOFB) • Pain

Ancillary Testing

- Ultrasound if the retina is not visible from dense vitreous inflammation to evaluate for retinal detachment, IOFB, and choroidal hemorrhage or effusion • CT for evaluation of an IOFB following trauma • Seidel testing of the bleb to evaluate for active leaking • Systemic evaluation with blood cultures to locate a primary source of infection when endogenous endophthalmitis is suspected • Vitreous and anterior chamber fluid samples obtained in the office or operating room should be sent to microbiology for gram stain, cultures, and sensitivities

Differential Diagnosis

- Phacoanaphylactic uveitis • Uveitis glaucoma hyphema syndrome • Isolated bleb infection • Pre-existing uveitis • Sympathetic uveitis

Treatment

- The Endophthalmitis Vitrectomy Study applies only to eyes within 6 weeks of cataract surgery
  - No formal controlled trials exist for the treatment of other forms of endophthalmitis
- Intravitreal injection of vancomycin (1 mg/0.1 mL) and ceftazidime (2.25 mg/0.1 mL) in bacterial infections
  - Amphotericin B (5 μg/0.1 mL) intravitreal injection is reserved for fungal endophthalmitis
- Pars plana vitrectomy with injection of antibiotics • Broad-spectrum topical antibiotics, prednisolone acetate 1%, and atropine 1% or scopolamine 0.25% after vitreous tap and injection of antibiotics
- Systemic antibiotics are essential for the treatment of endogenous endophthalmitis
  - The specific antibiotic used should be tailored to treat the offending agent
- Repeat injections of intravitreal antibiotics are given only if there are signs that the infection remains active and pain persists
  - Evidence of treated infection includes a reduction in the cellular response in the anterior chamber, clearing of the hypopyon, decrease in pain, decrease in lid edema, and resolution of the fibrin in the anterior chamber • Inflammation in the bleb and vitreous take longer to clear

Prognosis

- Visual acuity varies and depends on the extent of damage to the retina from infection, inflammation, or ocular trauma

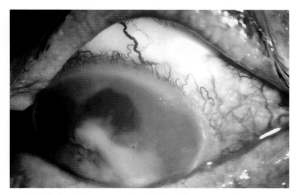

Fig. 13.10 A white, avascular bleb with surrounding conjunctival injection in bleb-associated endophthalmitis. Note the cornea edema and fibrin within the anterior chamber.

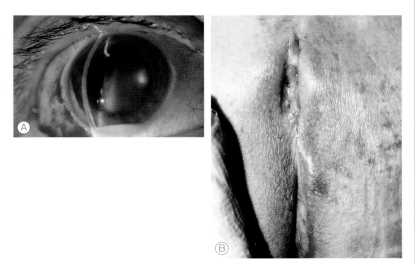

Fig. 13.11 A 56-year-old diabetic man presented with decreased vision secondary to endogenous endophthalmitis. (**A**) A hypopyon is present in the anterior chamber. (**B**) The source of the infection is a sacral abscess.

Neuroretinitis (Cat Scratch Disease)

Key Facts

- Caused by gram-negative bacilli (*Bartonella henselae*) spread by a cat scratch or bite
- Systemic symptoms include fever, malaise, and lymphadenopathy
- May be unilateral or bilateral
- No sexual or racial predilection

Clinical Findings

- Follicular conjunctivitis with regional lymphadenopathy
- Disc swelling
- Stellate macular exudate
- Chorioretinitis
- Vitreous cell
- Exudative retinal detachment
- Afferent pupillary defect in unilateral cases

Ancillary Testing

- Visual field shows a cecocentral scotoma
- B. henselae antibodies on serologic testing

Differential Diagnosis

- Hypertensive retinopathy
- Diabetic retinopathy with papillopathy
- Pseudotumor cerebri
- Sarcoidosis

Treatment

- Systemic antibiotics targeted at gram-negative organisms when ocular findings are severe and vision is affected
- In limited cases when vision is not affected, eyes may be closely observed

Prognosis

- Good visual prognosis in most cases

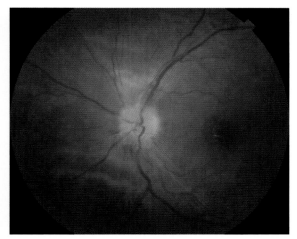

Fig. 13.12 Disc swelling with surrounding flame-shaped hemorrhages and early stellate macular exudate in an eye with neuroretinitis.

Fungal Endophthalmitis

Key Facts

- Common fungal etiologies include Candida (most common), Coccidioides, or Aspergillus
- Patients often present with pain and floaters
- Bilateral disease occurs in up to two-thirds of patients
- **History of:**
  - intravenous drug abuse • chronic indwelling intravenous catheter
    - septicemia treated with broad-spectrum intravenous antibiotics • solid organ transplantation

Clinical Findings

- Anterior uveitis
- Scleritis (rare finding)
- Vitreous cell
- Inflammatory vitreous opacities
- White, fluffy chorioretinal lesion
- Satellite chorioretinal lesions may be present
- Migration of the chorioretinal lesion through the retina into the vitreous cavity may occur

Ancillary Tests

- Fluorescein angiography shows staining of the chorioretinitis with early central hypofluorescence and a ring of hyperfluorescence or staining followed by complete staining of the entire lesion
- Ultrasound when vitreous inflammation prevents visualization of the retina
- Vitreous cultures with or without PCR
  - Positive vitreous cultures may be difficult to obtain—the organism often remains sequestered in the inflammatory mass
- Blood cultures
- Culture of the tips of any indwelling catheters or surgical wounds
- Consultation with an infectious disease specialist to utilize the most up-to-date systemic fungal treatments should be strongly considered

Differential Diagnosis

- Bacterial endophthalmitis
- Syphilis
- Tuberculosis
- Sarcoidosis
- Lymphoma

Treatment

- Systemic intravenous antifungal medications
- Intravitreal amphotericin B
- Intravitreal antibiotics to treat any underlying bacterial infection if the diagnosis of a fungal infection is unclear
- Pars plana vitrectomy for persistent vitreous inflammation and chorioretinal lesions
- Removal of any systemic indwelling catheters

Prognosis

- Visual outcome depends on extent of chorioretinitis and its proximity to the fovea

SECTION 13 • Infectious Diseases

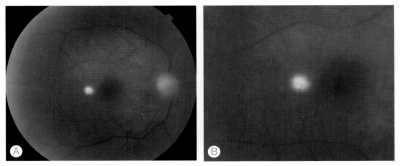

Fig. 13.13 White, circular subretinal infiltrate was identified in a 44-year-old man with blurred vision and acuity measuring 20/30. The patient had an indwelling intravenous catheter for antibiotic treatment of osteomyelitis and also has a history of intravenous drug abuse.

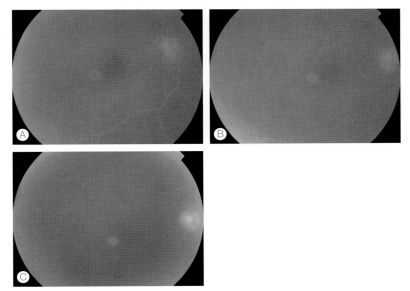

Fig. 13.14 (**A**) Fluorescein angiography shows early ring hyperfluorescence with central hypofluorescence. (**B,C**) Progressive staining of the entire lesion occurs in the later frames. Blood cultures were positive for Candida albicans.

Diffuse Unilateral Subacute Neuroretinitis

Key Facts

- Nematode infiltration of the retina • Exact subtype of the nematode is unknown • Retinal changes may be due to toxins excreted by the nematode • Usually unilateral, but bilateral cases have been described • Males affected more than females • Affects all age groups but most commonly occurs in second and third decades • Occurs more often in warmer climates in the southeastern USA and Caribbean

Clinical Findings

- Nematode may be identified in the subretinal space in an S-shaped or a coiled configuration • Focal yellow-white areas of chorioretinitis, which are transient and tend to occur only in the area of the nematode • Optic disc swelling (acute) • Anterior uveitis • Vitritis • Exudative retinal detachment • Depigmentation and mottling of the retinal pigment epithelium (RPE) (chronic) • Narrowing of retinal arterioles (chronic) • Afferent papillary defect (chronic) • Optic disc pallor (chronic) • Choroidal neovascularization or disciform scar formation (chronic) • Posterior subcapsular cataract (chronic)

Ancillary Tests

- Fluorescein angiography early in the disease process shows leakage from the optic disc and venous leakage
  - Active chorioretinitis shows hypofluorescence early with late hyperfluorescence • RPE changes inducing window defects are minimal at this juncture of the disease • Arteriovenous filling times may be delayed • As the disease progresses, window defect becomes more global, and delays in retinal and choroidal perfusion become more evident • Angiography is not useful in localizing the nematode
- The electroretinogram (ERG) is normal in the unaffected eye but shows increasing abnormalities as the retina becomes more involved
  - Advanced diffuse unilateral subacute neuroretinitis with chorioretinal scarring and atrophy may show an extinguished ERG
- Visual field may show central and paracentral field loss

Differential Diagnosis

- Sarcoidosis • Syphilis • Multifocal choroiditis with panuveitis • Acute posterior multifocal placoid pigment epitheliopathy • Serpiginous choroiditis • Toxoplasmosis • Ocular histoplasmosis syndrome • Retinitis pigmentosa

Treatment

- Laser photocoagulation of the nematode is the treatment of choice • Oral anthelmintic agents (thiabendazole or ivermectin) may be beneficial in eradicating the nematode • Pars plana vitrectomy with subretinal evacuation of the nematode

Prognosis

- Untreated disease over years leads to recurring disease with irreversible injury to the RPE and retina
  - Visual acuity in advanced forms of the disease leads to visual acuity that is 20/400 or worse
- Early treatment with eradication of the nematode before extensive destruction of the RPE and retina occurs may preserve useful visual acuity and prevent further vision loss

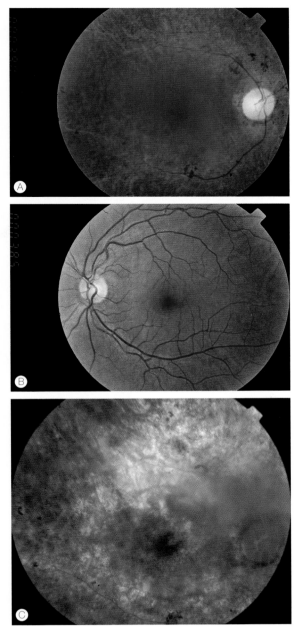

Fig. 13.15 (**A**) A 39-year-old woman from El Salvador with presumed chronic diffuse unilateral subacute neuroretinitis who noted progressive vision loss over a 13-year period that started soon after moving to the USA in 1981. (**B**) The retina of the left eye is normal. Electroretinogram was extinguished in the right eye but normal in the left eye. (**C**) Fluorescein angiography of the right eye shows global mottling of the RPE with window defect. The fluorescein angiogram of the left eye was normal.

Cysticercosis

Key Facts

- Rare disorder
- Occurs when humans ingest the eggs of the adult tapeworm Taenia solium
- The eggs hatch and the larvae of these eggs, cysticercus cellulosa, penetrate the intestinal wall and disseminate throughout the body, where they form cysts
- The posterior segment appears to be the most common location for ocular involvement

Clinical Findings

- Decreased visual acuity
- Translucent spherical cyst in the vitreous or subretinal space
- A single scolex is present and may be visible
- Vascular sheathing
- Retinal pigment epithelium alterations
- Non-rhegmatogenous retinal detachment
- Vitreous inflammation is present and intense when there is death of the cysticercus, otherwise the eye shows no inflammation

Ancillary Testing

- Ultrasound shows cyst with a centrally located scolex in the subretinal or preretinal space
- MRI or CT imaging of the brain may be considered to evaluate for central nervous system involvement

Differential Diagnosis

- Uveitis
- Intraocular foreign body

Treatment

- Observation if the visual acuity is poor and there is no intraocular inflammation
- Medical treatment for intraocular cysticercosis should be avoided—death of the organism leads to intense inflammation with eventual phthisis
- Pars plana vitrectomy for intravitreal cysticerci
- Subretinal cysticerci can be removed via pars plana vitrectomy or extraction through a sclerotomy

Prognosis

- Cysticerci may remain viable in the eye for about 2 years
- Death of the cysticercus causes intense inflammation
- Visual prognosis in most patients is poor

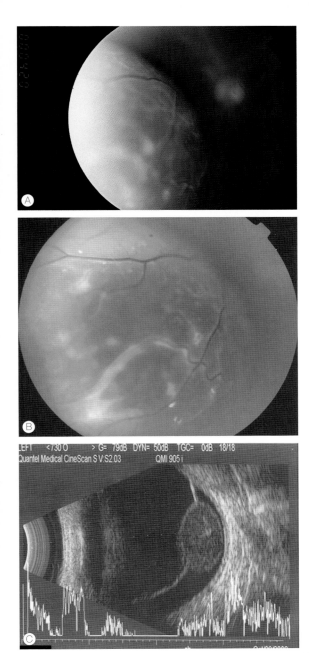

Fig. 13.16 (**A–C**) A patient from South America presented with a 2-year history of decreased vision to counting fingers in the left eye. A serous retinal detachment was present in the inferior nasal quadrant, with evidence of vasculitis (A,B). Ultrasound of the eye (**C**) showed a subretinal cystic structure with a retinal detachment consistent with a diagnosis of cysticercosis. The scolex is present in the center of the cystic space as a reverse shaped 'L'. (Courtesy of Caroline R. Baumal, MD.)

Syphilitic Chorioretinitis

Key Facts

- Infection with *Treponema pallidum*
- Sexually transmitted
- Increasing incidence over the past few decades with a rise in sexually transmitted diseases
- Ocular manifestations occur in secondary stage of syphilis
- Clinical findings of ocular syphilis are non-specific, hence the term 'the great masquerader'
- May be unilateral or bilateral

Clinical Findings

- Anterior uveitis
- Vitritis
- Vasculitis
- Focal areas of deep, yellow-white retinal infiltrates
- Disc edema
- Stellate maculopathy
- Optic atrophy (chronic)
- Chorioretinal atrophy (chronic)
- Pigment migration causing a salt and pepper fundus (chronic)

Ancillary Testing

- **Uveitis evaluation including:**
  - rapid plasma reagin • fluorescent treponemal antibody absorption assay • angiotensin-converting enzyme level • chest x-ray • purified protein derivative • CD4/HIV
- Consultation with primary care physician or infectious disease specialist for further systemic evaluation and treatment options

Differential Diagnosis

- Acute retinal necrosis
- Progressive outer retinal necrosis
- Cytomegalovirus retinitis
- Sarcoid uveitis
- Tuberculosis
- Toxoplasmosis chorioretinitis
- Serpiginous choroidopathy
- Acute posterior multifocal placoid pigment epitheliopathy

Treatment

- Topical prednisolone acetate 1% for anterior uveitis
- Penicillin G intravenous or intramuscular
- Doxycycline, erythromycin, ceftriaxone, and ampicillin may be substituted for patients allergic to penicillin
- Oral corticosteroids may be considered for concomitant scleritis and optic neuritis but should be used only in conjunction with antibiotics

Prognosis

- T. pallidum rapidly responds to penicillin G
  - Prompt recognition and treatment will lead to full visual recovery
- Untreated, chronic syphilitic uveitis will lead to chorioretinal atrophy, optic disc atrophy, persistent intraocular inflammation, and diminished visual acuity

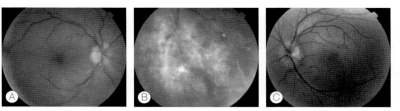

Fig. 13.17 A 28-year-old man was diagnosed with HIV and syphilitic chorioretinitis. (A) A red-free photograph shows focal areas of vitreous inflammatory balls attached to the posterior hyaloid overlying the temporal macula and superior temporal vascular arcade. (B) Vasculitis and punctate areas of chorioretinitis present in the inferior retina. (C) Disc edema was the only clinical sign of infection in the left eye and was more prominent than the disc swelling seen in the right eye (A).

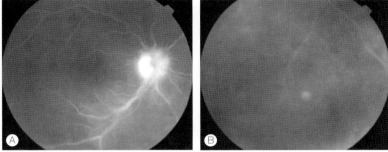

Fig. 13.18 Fluorescein angiography from the right eye of the patient in Fig. 13.20 shows leakage from the disc (A), vessels, and inflammatory infiltrate (B).

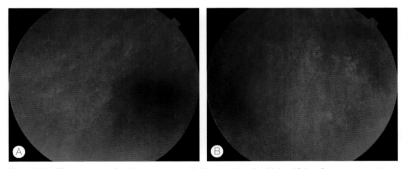

Fig. 13.19 The areas of active chorioretinitis resolved within 48 h after treatment with intravenous penicillin G and now visible as areas of chorioretinal atrophy (A,B), 6 weeks post treatment.

Toxocariasis

Key Facts

- Caused by *Toxocara canis*
- T. canis is spread through contaminated soil or exposure to infected puppies
- ≤10% of a population may be infected with T. canis
- The organism is ingested and produces larvae that migrate to end organs, in which they encyst

Clinical Findings

- White granuloma in the posterior pole or peripheral retina represents encysted larvae
- Vitreous bands
- Retinal folds that often extend to the optic disc

Ancillary Testing

- *T. canis* titers

Differential Diagnosis

- Retinoblastoma
- Pars planitis
- Sarcoidosis
- Persistent fetal vasculature
- Familial exudative vitreoretinopathy
- Coats disease
- Retinopathy of prematurity

Treatment

- Observation
- Pars plana vitrectomy to treat macular folds may be considered.

Prognosis

- Poor visual prognosis if a falciform fold is present in the macula

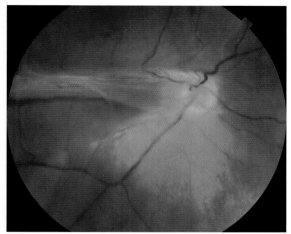

Fig. 13.20 A falciform fold of the retina in the macula of a patient with counting fingers vision from toxocariasis. A granuloma was present in the temporal peripheral retina. Toxicariasis titers were positive.

Fundus flavimaculata (Stargardt disease), 194–197
Fungal endophthalmitis, 268–269

G

Ganciclovir implant, 254, 255
Geographic atrophy, age-related macular degeneration, 14, 15
Giant cell arteritis, 38, 40, 42, 44
Glaucoma
  angle closure
    persistent fetal vasculature, 80
    posterior scleritis, 240
    Vogt–Koyanagi–Harada syndrome, 242
  choroidal hemorrhage, 154
  neovascular
    central retinal artery obstruction, 42, 45
    central retinal vein occlusion, 36
    Coats disease, 46
    familial exudative vitreopathy, 78
    ocular ischemic syndrome, 62
    proliferative diabetic retinopathy, 6, 10
    radiation retinopathy, 52
  post-surgical cystoid macular edema, 176
Gyrate atrophy, 206–207

H

Haemophilus influenzae endophthalmitis, 264
Hamartoma
  combined retina/retinal pigment epithelium, 126–129
  retinal astrocytic, 105, 136
Harada disease, 152
Hard exudates, non-proliferative diabetic retinopathy, 2, 3, 4, 5
Hemangioma
  choroidal, 116–117
  retinal capillary, 130–133
  retinal cavernous, 134–135
Hematologic disorders, 72–73
Hemoglobinopathies, 42
Herpes simplex virus, acute retinal necrosis, 252
Histoplasma capsulatum, 234
HIV disease
  cytomegalovirus retinitis, 254, 255
  progressive outer retinal necrosis, 250, 251
  retinopathy, 70–71
  syphilitic chorioretinitis, 275

HLA-A29, 230
HLA-B5, 246
Homocystinuria, 38, 90, 142
Hydroxychloroquine toxicity, 184–185
Hypercortisolism, 178
Hyperlipidemia, 2, 38
Hypertension, 2, 32, 36, 38, 52, 64, 72, 152, 154
Hypertensive retinopathy, 58–61
  cystoid macular edema, 176
  macular hole, 170
Hyphema
  choroidal rupture, 96
  intraocular foreign body, 92
  retinoblastoma, 106
Hypopyon
  Behçet disease, 246
  endophthalmitis
    cataract surgery-associated, 260
    endogenous, 264, 265
Hypotony
  chorioretinal folds, 166
  proliferative vitreoretinopathy, 150

I

Idiopathic choroidal neovascularization, 20–21
Idiopathic juxtafoveal telangiectasia, 50–51
Indwelling catheters, 264, 268, 269
Infectious diseases, 250–277
Inflammatory disorders, 240–247
Intracranial hemorrhage
  child abuse, 82
  Terson syndrome, 68, 69
Intracranial retinoblastoma, 108
Intraocular lymphoma, 120–121
Intraretinal fluid
  angioid streaks, 26
  idiopathic choroidal neovascularization, 20
  neovascular age-related macular degeneration, 16
  ocular histoplasmosis syndrome, 234
Intraretinal hemorrhage
  acute retinal necrosis, 253
  cilioretinal artery occlusion with central retinal vein occlusion, 40
  cystoid macular edema, 176
  cytomegalovirus retinitis, 254, 255
  familial exudative vitreopathy, 78
  hematologic disorders, 72, 73
  idiopathic choroidal neovascularization, 20
  Purtscher's retinopathy, 66
  radiation retinopathy, 52

Index

Index

S

Index